THE HEALTHY EXECUTIVE

The Daily Telegraph

THE HEALTHY EXECUTIVE

Dr. R. M. Youngson

Published by Telegraph Publications,
135 Fleet Street, London EC4P 4BL

© Telegraph Publications/William Curtis Ltd

Whilst every care has been taken to ensure the accuracy
of the contents of this work, no responsibility of loss
occasioned to any person acting or refraining from
action as a result of any statement in it can be
accepted.

Typeset by BSC Print, London

Printed in Great Britain by Biddles Ltd

British Library Cataloguing in Publication Data
Youngson, R.M.
   The healthy executive.
   1. Executives – Health programs
   1. Title
   613 RA776.5

   ISBN 0-86367-189-6
   ISBN 0-86367-180-2 Pbk

Contents

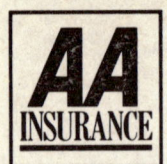 AUTOMOBILE ASSOCIATION

PROTECTION AND INVESTMENT PLANNING LTD

Registered as an authorised, independent intermediary as required by the Financial Services Act to provide impartial advice on life insurance, savings plans, investment bonds, unit trusts, pensions and mortgages.

Recommendations are made from the best products available across the market.

For further information please complete the coupon below or telephone our Helpline on 0256-493139

Registered Office: Fanum House, Basingstoke, Hampshire, RG21 2EA.
Registered in England Number 2023217

PLEASE SEND MORE DETAILS . . .

☐ Family Protection Insurance   ☐ Disability Insurance

☐ Medical Insurance   ☐ Regular Savings

☐ Mortgages   ☐ Pensions

☐ Investments   ☐ Unit Trusts

Name_____

Address_____

_____

Date of Birth_____Smoker/Non Smoker (delete as appropriate)

Return to: AA Protection & Investment Planning Ltd.,
PO Box 74, Basingstoke, Hampshire RG21 2EA.

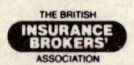

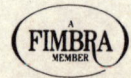

Introduction

Health has become a vital commodity in the economics of modern business and administrative life. Good executives are expensive, and firms who have made a large investment in them, expect the investment to pay off. So the next time the managing director greets you with a hearty 'How are you, my dear fellow?' bear in mind that his concern is not exclusively for your welfare. He is also concerned about the duration of your effectiveness as a highly programmed executive machine. He is interested in your MTBF – mean time between failures. As he grasps your hand, gives you that famous piercing look and says, 'You seem very fit, old boy!' he may well be thinking, 'Fine! Smith looks as if he might be able to keep up the good work for another year or two'.

When you suffer your coronary there will, no doubt, be many expressions of sympathy to you (or to your grieving spouse) but there will also be a certain amount of ire. The firm will carry on somehow and, in due course, someone will take your place. Your fellow executives will, however, know that your self-indulgence, smoking, physical idleness, or whatever it was that finally led to the clogging up of your coronary artery, was an expensive luxury for the business which will take a long time to amortize.

It is now recognised that, only too often, top people are depreciating hardware and very expensive hardware at that. The software – call it education, work experience or programming, as you will – is also very costly. In today's fast moving environment it rapidly declines in value if it is not constantly updated and it may even develop bugs. Too often, senior executives and administrators are unable to meet the challenge of change and innovation. Rigidity of outlook, rejection of new methods and philosophies and a refusal to think expansively, can almost invariably be attributed to a decline in physical or mental health. The standard theory, that it is natural for energy and flexibility of mind and body to decline with age, is on a par with the equally widely held fallacy that it is natural and normal to get heavier as you get older.

Now it would be unreasonable to expect disinterested concern for the work ethic to be foremost in your motivation. If it is – congratulations! It is more likely that you are concerned about your health mainly because of its bearing on *you* and, in particular, on your continuing effectiveness as a human being. You will have perceived already that disease and disability are to be feared, not so much for their intrinsic unpleasantness, as for their effect on our capacity to live life to the full. This, of course, includes the ability to work hard, effectively, competitively and successfully.

Now it is possible that for some of you reading this book, the message has come very late, perhaps too late. For some, the effects of years of systematic self-inflicted injury may already be so severe as to be irremediable. For those who are more fortunate, however, one of the central lessons to be learned from a book such as this is that the adaptation the body makes to certain sustained forms of abuse is not only irreversible, but is exceedingly damaging to the quality of future life. We are talking about permanent tissue and organ changes imperceptibly brought about, over the years, by defective and unnatural patterns of living. The body is wonderfully adaptable and will tolerate punishment to an astonishing degree, but eventually irremediable alterations occur. The purpose of this book therefore is to brief you on the nature of these risks in order to give you the chance to avoid them. Or, at least, to give you the chance to add nothing further to the existing burden of destructive change.

You may ask what evidence exists for the assertion that certain patterns of life are unnatural? A knowledge of human physiology (body function) viewed in the context of biological evolution has brought about a consensus of opinion, which now predominates in informed medical circles. This view is that, as the present form and function of our bodies evolved so that we should be able to survive in a hostile physical environment, the use of the body in a manner normal for such an environment is 'natural' and will tend towards its well-being. We can nowadays, if we wish, enjoy the luxury of living as natural men and women while, at the same time, avoiding most of the hazards which caused the life of primitive man to be brutish and short. Unfortunately, the advances of civilisation which make it easy for us to avoid these hazards, also make it easy to avoid many of the apparent discomforts whose side effects are, in fact, health-giving.

Looked at in this way, it is natural to walk long distances, to run when necessary and often to get breathless, to be regularly short of food, to stay thin and to be frequently tired. It is hardly necessary to enlarge on the list of behavioural patterns which, viewed in evolutionary terms, are only too obviously unnatural.

So, as responsible people, we cannot ignore health matters and we cannot escape the conclusion that something radical must be done. Maintenance contracts are fine for desk-top micros and, to a limited extent, may be of value to people as well. With people, however, the matter is not so simple and, managerial concern notwithstanding, basically depends almost entirely on the individual – you.

What is to be done? Well, that is what this book is all about. It is about longevity and about the quality of life, for longevity must be more than mere survival. The stroke victim and the cardiac or respiratory cripple may cling frantically to life, but in many cases such life is a mere humiliating dependency. For some the restrictions and limitations and their resulting frustration, make mere existence so painful that they would gladly accept the abbreviation such disorders normally effect. So this book is not primarily concerned with prolongation of life, nor is it simply about the avoidance of disease.

Health is much more than just the absence of disease. Nor is it, as is often thought, a property of the physical body alone. Health is a positive state of mind, body and attitude – an outgoing, motivating state compounded of a sense of well-being, optimism and a desire to be doing or creating. It expresses itself in a strong inclination for work, a proper regard for one's own worth and a respect and concern for others. It implies the existence of values and standards.

The word 'health' literally means 'wholeness' and derives from an Old English word related to the verb 'to heal' – ie 'to make whole'. The Greeks had two words for health, 'hygeia' meaning 'a good way of living' and 'euexia' meaning 'a good habit of body'. Therefore being well in body requires that we establish good habits of living, for we, as individuals, are to a large extent responsible for the state of our own health.

Ill-health can turn people in upon themselves, focusing their attention on their own miseries at the expense of concern for others. It is often a state of supreme selfishness. The relationship between body and mind is so close that the separation of mutual cause and effect is often difficult and sometimes impossible. This is most apparent in the motivation behind the way in which we commonly abuse our bodies and in doing so effect, by our own act, the major causes of disease and ill-health today. No one reading a book of this kind can be unaware that body abuse by physical and mental idleness, overeating, smoking, excess alcohol intake, improper habits of work and relaxation, can be gravely damaging to our health and happiness. Yet many will have to admit to this kind of body abuse.

Why do we do it? Why, for instance, do we eat so much? Is self-gratification, the need for self-reward, perhaps for consolation, so important that we indulge it, fully aware that gluttony will not only spoil our sexual attractiveness, but may even kill us?

Another important enemy of health is mind abuse. By this

we mean the cultivation of anger, hatred, jealousy, spiteful-
ness, prejudice – all activities which, like body abuse, seem
at the time to be gratifying. But they are all damaging, even
destructive, to our health and happiness and to the quality of
our lives.

Cause and prevention of disease

A great deal is now known about the factors leading to ill
health or premature death. Heart disease, cancer of the lung,
cerebral thrombosis and many others are well understood
and any reasonable individual can eliminate the known risk
factors. Yet, in spite of this, the death rate from these conditions not only remains high, but is actually rising.

The number of people who died from coronary thrombosis in Britain in 1968 was 138,569, but ten years later in
1978, deaths totalled 160,458. That is nearly 22,000 extra,
unnecessary deaths. In England alone in 1980 some 144,080
people died from this cause. In the same year the figure for
deaths from cancer of the lung was 33,327 – another horrifying increase on previous figures. Deaths from alcohol-
caused cirrhosis of the liver rose, during the same period, by
20 per cent in women and 30 per cent in men.

The causes of all these unnecessary deaths are known. The
means of prevention are known. Yet, everywhere people are
killing themselves or so damaging their health that their lives
are going to be both miserable and shorter. Most people
behave in this reckless way because the only way they seem
able to learn is by bitter experience. Unfortunately, these are
the people to whom learning comes, if it ever does, too late.
People capable of learning and understanding also behave in
this way and the only explanation would seem to be that the
advice received has been insufficiently explicit. A situation
this book hopes to remedy.

It does not purport to be a universal panacea. You will find
no wonder cures, fancy diets or 'alternative medicine'. What
you will get is hard, uncompromising advice based on established scientific fact, advice which will not always be easy to

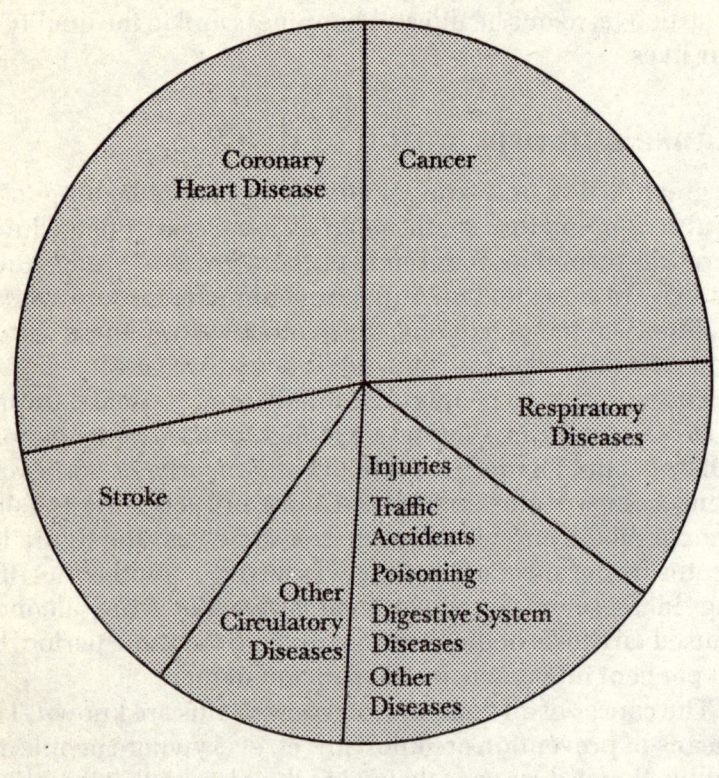

Figure 1 —
Breakdown of major causes of death in England and Wales 1985

take but which you ignore at your peril. You will not be faced with a list of prohibitions of all the things that seem to make life pleasant. What you will get are clear explanations of the causes and means of prevention of the major diseases, and a great deal of valuable guidance on how to develop a positive approach to health and happiness.

The seven rules of physical health

Attempts have been made, scientifically, to try and find out whether observance of certain rules of conduct can actually be relied upon to lead to a genuine improvement in health. This study, at the University College of Los Angeles School of Public Health, began by investigating the effects of various health practices derived from the observation of the behaviour of people in a high state of physical vigour and enjoying long life. As a result of these studies, they came up with a set of seven 'rules' for good health. When they studied the effects of conforming to these rules, this is what they found. People who observed all seven rules were found to be healthier and to live longer than those who obeyed only six; those who conformed to six did better than those who obeyed only five; and so on right down the scale.

Some of the findings were remarkable. For instance, the physical condition of those people over 75 who obeyed all seven rules, was equal to that of people aged 40 who obeyed only one or two of the rules. People who conformed to six or all seven rules had a life expectancy 11 years longer, at the age of 45, than people who obeyed only three or less.

By now you are probably agog to know what the 'rules' are. Well, they are rather mundane, but none the less important for that. They are:

(1) Eat breakfast.
(2) Do not eat between meals.
(3) Keep your weight down.
(4) Do not smoke cigarettes.
(5) Drink only in moderation.

(6) Take exercise every day.

(7) Get seven hours of sleep every night.

Quite a proportion of this book is devoted to helping you to conform to these excellent rules.

There are many other factors which affect health, of course – things such as heredity, susceptibility to disease, the misfortune of accidental injury and so on – but these seven rules are matters over which you have complete control and which you are free to observe or to disregard as you wish. The purpose of this book is to provide you not only with rational grounds for making the decision to conform to these rules, but also with strong motivation to do so.

As already stressed, physical health has a major bearing on mental and social health. But we need to ensure that the process has an adequate chance to work in the opposite direction also. Later in the book you will therefore, be introduced to some rules of psychosocial health. These, with their direct bearing on personal relationships and consequently personal happiness, have a major part to play in promoting health in the widest sense.

However the merits of longevity may be qualified, we all crave it. So, let us take a look at the question of life-span.

How long do we have?

Most people think that the human life span is extending, but this is not so. There is no indication that the natural span – about 100 years – is lengthening. What is happening is that people are living longer and getting near to, or reaching, the normal upper age limit. Life expectancy is increasing because medical and technological advances are enabling more people to avoid death before reaching the full span.

In privileged western societies, deaths in early years are becoming less common and for the first time in history, most people can look forward with reasonable confidence to growing old. This is a new phenomenon for mankind. Two thousand years ago, the average life span in Greece and Rome – the most civilised parts of the world – was about 22 years. In England, in the Middle Ages, it was about 33 years and around 1850 it had risen to only 40 years. By 1900 the average life span was close to 50 years and today it is over 70 years.

So what are the factors preventing us from achieving our full natural life span? It is not much help to look at the causes of death in the Middle Ages, or even at the end of the nineteenth century. In those days the one great killer was infection and, violent death apart, nearly everyone died from diseases like pneumonia, septicaemia (blood poisoning), tuberculosis, cholera, plague, malaria and so on. People simply did not live long enough to develop the conditions which are the major causes of death today – heart disease, hypertension (high blood pressure), stroke, kidney and liver failure, and cancer.

Today, infection as a major cause of death, has been virtually eliminated. The *Penicillium notatum* spore that floated in through the window of Alexander Fleming's laboratory in 1928 and landed on a culture plate of Staphylococcus, has had astonishing consequences. Penicillin and later antibiotics have given us the means of controlling almost every known infection and the whole aspect of individual health has changed. An entirely new group of diseases has taken the ascendency.

It has been estimated that if the one major killer group – diseases of the heart and circulation – could be completely eliminated, life expectancy would rise by no less than 12 years. In other words, the present average life span would rise to 85. Cancer has a much smaller effect and its total elimination would raise the average span by only about two years. Well below cancer come causes like traffic and domestic accidents, then lung disease and diabetes.

What is ageing?

What is it that puts the limit of around one hundred years on our life span? Our bodies are composed of living cells, many of which are constantly reproducing themselves so that tissue damage from wear and tear may be repaired. This process of replication is going on all the time in our bodies, the cells in the reproductive organs, and those subject to most wear and tear (such as those of the skin or the lining of the bowel) requiring the most frequent division.

It is not difficult to arrange suitable nutrition for cells, so that they can be made to survive and reproduce themselves outside the body. 'Tissue cultures' of this type are now commonplace. So long as the conditions of nutrition are satisfied, the cell culture will continue to grow without limit. But the cells of such artificial cultures are abnormal and are incapable of the many important functions required of healthy cells within the body. They are, in fact cancer cells and all they can do is grow and reproduce.

When normal cells are cultured, it is found that there is a definite limit to the number of times they can reproduce. This number has been repeatedly checked in different trials. Cells from a foetus or young baby will double in number between 40 and 60 times and the culture will then die. The average of 50 population doublings is remarkably constant. However, if cells are taken from a middle aged man and cultured, the number of doublings before the cells die will be reduced to about 25. Trials have shown that the limiting factor is not the donor's age but solely the number of times the cells reproduce. Even keeping the cells in suspended animation by freezing for several years does not alter this fact.

They will just resume where they left off, undergo the immutable 50 or so doublings, then die. Cells from a wide range of human donors, of ages from birth to 90 years, show a steady average decrease in the number of times they reproduce before the culture dies.

This principle of 50 cell population doublings does seem to put a definite limit on our life expectancy. However, this does not imply that, barring accidents or disease, we will all live until our cells just stop dividing. In fact, more than 100 different changes in the structure and function of cells have been noted, long before they lose the ability to replicate. These changes, which increase progressively as the number of cell divisions is used up, progressively impair the cell's ability to perform its proper functions. It is these changes which produce all the well-known signs of old age and which result in the death of the individual long before the cells cease to divide.

Do we want to live longer?

Considerable research has been directed to the study of these cell changes, in the hope of being able to arrest them and prolong life. But do we really want to live longer than the 'allotted span' – which is now 100 years?

Certainly, age changes being what they are at present, it is doubtful whether there would be much point in it. The question has been put to many elderly people, all of them in possession of their faculties, and the general opinion is against undue prolongation. That view may, of course, be a reflection of the natural ability which most old people have to view their approaching demise with a remarkable degree of acceptance. Were it possible to slow the rate of cell ageing, the outlook of a well-preserved person of 90 might come to resemble that of a contemporary man or woman in the prime of life. But, at the present stage of medical advance, and accepting the inevitable physical deterioration of age, we might do well to be content with the present normal span, and think ourselves lucky if we reach it.

1   The body as a machine

This chapter contains a straight-forward account of what you need to know about how your body functions, if the rest of the book is going to make sense. The mechanistic view of life, which has predominated throughout this century, proposes that all bodily phenomena, however complex, can effectively be described in terms of physical and chemical processes. All the data so far derived from proper observation and experiment support this view. The body is a machine – amazingly complex – but a machine all the same.

An outline understanding of the structure and function of the body should be part of your mental equipment. Without such knowledge your chances of running into health problems are increased and you are ill-equipped to look critically at the many references to medical matters in the news and information media.

One useful way of considering the body is to start from an awareness of the central importance of the brain. This organ is the seat of all personal satisfaction, intelligence, memory and emotion as well as the coordinator and initiator of all body activity. The brain must be regarded as the essential component for which the rest of the body acts as a vehicle. It is constantly receiving an immense amount of input data, most of it below conscious level, from a great many sensory receptors and is continuously correlating this data (which comes from both the outside world and from the rest of the body) with previously stored information.

As a result of this massive information input, the brain is prompted to initiate intention and action. To fulfil intention, the brain must act through a system external to itself. That system must be capable of movement, interaction, feeding, communication and sensory stimulation of all kinds.

There are 12 pairs of major nerves that emerge directly from the brain (the 'cerebrum') and go to the nose (olfactory nerves), the eyes (optic nerves and eye-moving nerves), the skin and muscles of the face, the ears (acoustic nerves), the tongue, the muscles of the neck and the heart and bowels. In addition, the stalk of the brain carries major nerve trunks down the inside of the spine, from whence these nerves emerge at all levels to supply messages to, and obtain information from, all the muscles and sense receptors of the body. Input data is correlated in various discrete microprocessors in various parts of the brain and, as a result, the brain is able to exert precise controlling influence on every part of the body.

In addition to the nerve connections, the brain also exerts control by means of chemical substances called 'hormones' (literally, 'wanderers') which it releases into the bloodstream and which are carried all around the body to exert their effect wherever there are receptors capable of responding to them.

Before moving on from the brain, we should mention that this amazing structure is surrounded by a layer of cushioning fluid, then some tough membranes and finally is totally enclosed in a very strong bone container which is mounted high up and out of harm's way. In this way the brain is excellently protected and would come to little harm were we not, apparently, determined to put it to the maximum danger possible by indulging in activities like heavy drinking and high-speed motorway driving in poor weather conditions.

The function of locomotion

The body's locomotive system is amazingly well-designed and wonderfully adapted for carrying the brain around. The skeletal system of the body is articulated by ball and socket joints (hips and shoulders), hinge and rotating joints (knees and elbows) and cushion, shock-absorbed joints (spine). These joints are stabilised and secured by tough, ingeniously contrived ligaments and fibrous capsules. Operating across both sides of each of these joints are groups of muscles so disposed as to enable the joints (at least in youth and health) to go through their full range of movement.

The muscles, which comprise about half the total body weight, consist of large collections of protein fibres bound up in fibrous sheaths. Muscles are shaped according to their function and to their attachments. When the brain sends a message to any particular muscle group, by way of the 'motor' nerves, the muscle on one side of the joint will shorten while those on the other side will smoothly let out slack. In this way the joint will flex and the required movement will be achieved.

Locomotion is a complex mechanical process, calling for remarkable timing in the contraction of a great many different muscle groups. Many muscles will be acting to brace or balance one part of the skeleton so as to allow another part to move relative to the first. Almost all the voluntary muscles of the body are involved in the act of walking, and although many of them may, at any one moment, be engaged simply in holding some part of the body steady, they have to perform work in doing so.

Such a complex function requires a real-time computer for its control and this is provided by a sort of subsidiary brain, called the cerebellum, which hangs down underneath the back of the cerebrum. The cerebellum gets input from the cerebrum to tell it what movements are intended. But it also gets input from the eyes, from the position sensors (the 'semicircular canals') in the inner ears and from all the voluntary muscles of the body. These various inputs inform the cerebellum about the position of the head relative to the body, and about the position of all the limbs. Having put all that information together the cerebellum works out which muscles must be contracted to achieve the desired movement. This somewhat abbreviated account will give you some idea of the complexity of brain function needed to carry out what may, at first sight, seem to be quite a simple function.

The size of individual muscles is determined almost entirely by the amount of physical work that they are called upon to do. Sustained, hard muscular work will ensure that, within the limits of the size and strength of the skeleton, large, healthy muscles are produced. Such work will also ensure that the function of the lungs and of the heart reaches a high degree of efficiency ('fitness') so that heavy work can be undertaken without difficulty. There is really no substitute for this kind of conditioning, especially in youth and early adult life, and to undertake it is a splendid investment for the future. Children and young people who, for one reason or another, do not undertake regular hard physical exercise are unlikely fully to compensate for it later in life.

The physical capacity of our body soon adapts itself to the amount of physical work we do. So, if we want to keep it capable of work, then the only way is to go on working it throughout life. So you should never miss an opportunity for exercise, the effects and benefits of which are dealt with in more detail in Chapter 9.

The outward shape of the body depends firstly on the proportions of the skeleton, secondly on the shape, proportion and bulk of the muscles, thirdly on the thickness of the layer of fat covering the muscles and finally on the bulk of the fat deposits in the abdomen.

The fuel supply

Like any other machine that does work, the body requires a supply of energy in the form of chemical fuel. However, the body goes one further and incorporates a chemical processing plant which can accept input from a surprising variety of different fuels. So long as these conform to the general description of 'food', the body does not mind too much. As you will learn in Chapter 8, all food is broken down in the digestive system into three simpler chemical substances of which one, glucose, is the basic fuel of the body.

The body needs a lot of glucose as this is constantly being

burned up and converted to carbon dioxide and water, in order to release chemical energy for muscle contraction, nerve impulse production and the maintenance of body temperature. We are accustomed to the idea of fuels, such as petrol, being burned at high temperatures. For non-biological machines, fuels which oxidise at high temperatures are most useful as they can give off their energy very quickly. If certain chemical activators called 'enzymes' are present, however, oxidation can occur at much lower temperatures and that is what happens in the body.

The oxygen supply

Oxidation (burning) can occur only in the presence of oxygen and this constitutes about 20 per cent of the atmospheric air. Oxygen is our most urgent need. If we are deprived of oxygen for even a few minutes we will die. When a cardiac arrest occurs in hospital the first thing done is to check the time. A supply of oxygen to the brain must be provided within a very few minutes or permanent, serious damage will be done.

Every cell in the body needs a constant supply of oxygen and it is important to understand how this feat is accomplished. The greater part of the chest cavity is occupied by the two lungs. These are rather like a pair of bellows, containing hundreds of thousands of tiny air sacs, all communicating by means of branching trees of tubes, with the nose and mouth and, through them, with the outside air. The chest cavity is air-tight and by virtue of the way in which the ribs can spread outwards and upwards and the diaphragm can flatten downwards, the inside volume of this cavity during breathing is capable of great expansion. Because the lungs are elastic this increase in volume during the expansion phase, means that new air will be sucked in to fill the tiny air sacs, only to be expelled again when the volume of the chest returns to normal.

Now the moist walls of the tiny air sacs are also the walls of millions of very small blood vessels called 'capillaries' which are the ultimate branches of the large arteries carrying

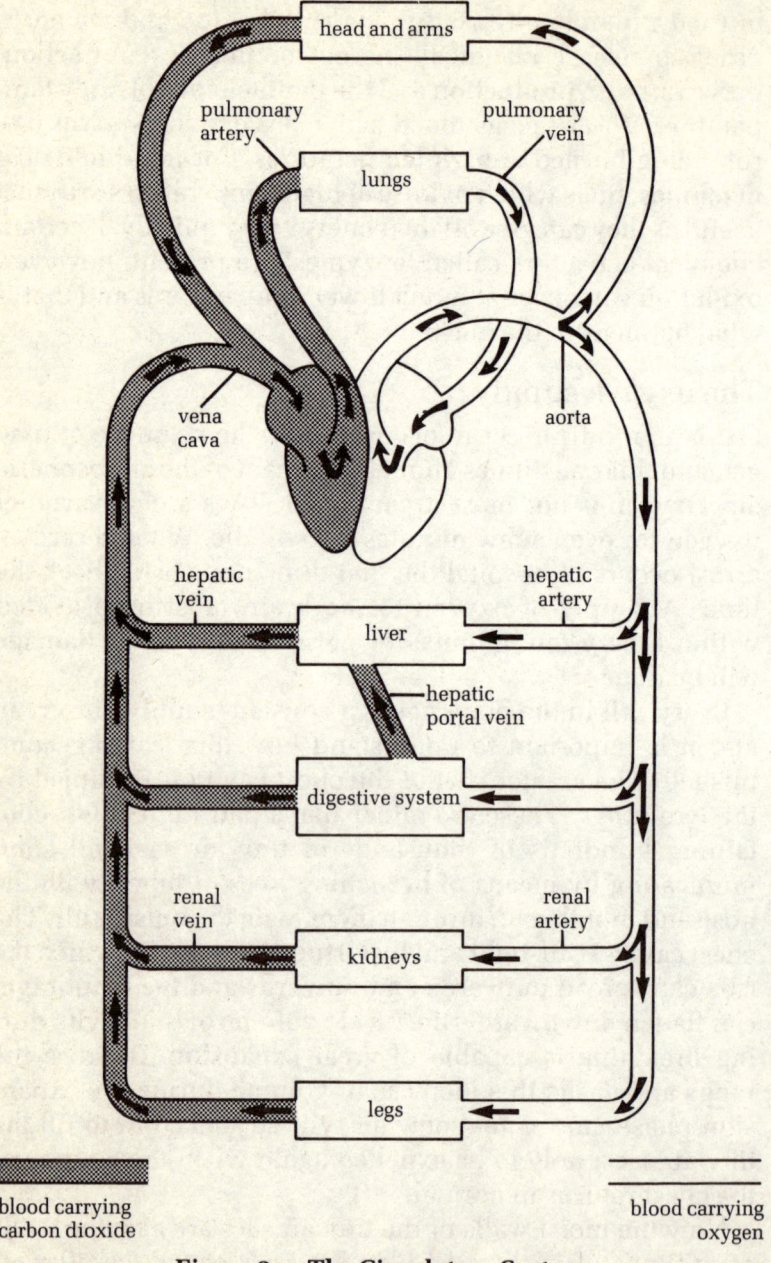

blood carrying
carbon dioxide

blood carrying
oxygen

Figure 2 — The Circulatory System

blood to the lungs from the heart. In this way, a considerable quantity of blood is spread out over a very large total surface area and is brought into intimate contact with the oxygen. Each cubic millimeter of blood contains about five million red cells and each of these cells is filled with a remarkable compound of iron and protein called haemoglobin. Haemoglobin has the property of linking up with oxygen, if its environment is rich in oxygen, and of giving up oxygen if its environment is low in oxygen. So when blood passes through the lungs the haemoglobin automatically picks up oxygen and when it passes through tissues which are short of oxygen, it is released.

So as to fulfil this purpose the blood must circulate, just like the water in a central-heating plant. Just as a central-heating installation needs a pump to keep the water going round, so does the blood circulation. In this case, the pump is known as the heart and that is all the heart does. It is really a double pump, one side pumping blood to the lungs and back to the other side. This side then pumps the newly oxygenated blood from the lungs all around the body and into the head. Blood, now short of oxygen, returns from the head and body by way of the veins and enters the side of the pump connected at the lungs. The heart is made of solid muscle of a special type which contracts spontaneously, and the blood is directed by means of very efficient one-way valves within and at the outlet of the heart. The heart beats about 70 times a minute and that is over 2,000 million times a year, so it is a fairly reliable pump, bearing in mind that most hearts keep working for 70 years or more.

In order to do all this work the heart muscle, of course, needs a pretty good oxygen and glucose supply of its own. In fact, it gets priority, for the very first branches of the main artery coming out of the left side of the heart (the aorta) run back into the heart muscle itself.

These branches form a sort of crown over the heart and, for this reason, are called the 'coronary' arteries. It is hardly necessary to stress that the coronary arteries are very important and you will find a good deal of reference to them in this book. The fact that some 160,000 people die in the UK each year through failure of their coronary arteries will give you some idea of the extent of this particular problem.

The digestive system

Diet and nutrition are major subjects in this book and it is important for you to have some idea of the background to this topic. Those of you regularly involved in entertaining clients will find the additional information contained in Chapter 8 even more beneficial.

The digestive system consists of a tube, about 25 feet long, which starts at the mouth and terminates at the rectum. The processing of food starts with the cutting and grinding action of the teeth, the lubrication with saliva and the beginning of the biochemical breakdown with the action of the first 'enzyme'. Food meets a variety of digestive enzymes on its way down the gut. Although these act on different types of food, they all act in a similar way to break the food down chemically, into simpler materials.

Food passes along the tube by a process called 'peristalsis' in which the circular muscles of the tube wall relax in front of the lump of food and contract behind it. This action forces the food to slide along the tube and is, of course, essential, if the tube is not to get blocked. When peristalsis becomes disordered and acts against itself we get severe colic.

Food passes from the mouth down the gullet to the stomach, a muscular bag where the food is further digested by stomach acid and enzyme. It then passes down into the duodenum where bile from the liver (see page 27) and more enzymes from the pancreas, attack it. Soon it is in a fit state to be absorbed through the wall of the small intestine and practically all the material of food value is indeed absorbed.

The residue, mostly cellulose, now passes on into the large intestine (colon) and there excess water is absorbed. The resulting material, which consists of the unabsorbable remains of whatever has been eaten and a large number of bacteria, is eventually excreted.

The liver

This is the largest organ in the body and fills the upper part of the abdomen on the right side, under the diaphragm. All the blood in the body passes through it, and in addition to the normal arterial supply, a second major inflow of blood occurs from the veins draining the intestines. These veins carry sugars, fats, amino acids, vitamins and other substances from digested food which have been absorbed through the wall of the small intestine. The liver takes up all these raw materials and gets to work on them, converting them into forms which the rest of the body can use. The main fuel, glucose, is stored in the liver in a concentrated form called glycogen, and a number of other essential substances, including most of the vitamins, are also stored there. This, however, is not all it does.

Fats, in the form in which they occur in the diet, are not readily usable by the body because they will not mix with water. This problem is overcome by means of a liquid called bile, which is formed in the liver and passed down the 'bile duct' into the bowel where it comes into contact with the fat which has been eaten. Bile is a sort of detergent or emulsifying agent and under its influence, fats are broken down into tiny globules to form a kind of milk which is easily absorbed. In addition to the bile salts which make the fats water-soluble, the fluid contains a considerable quantity of brown pigment called bilirubin. Any obstruction to the outflow of bile into the gut leads to the accumulation of this in the bloodstream where it gets deposited in the skin causing the condition we know as jaundice.

One of the main functions of the liver is to render toxic substances harmless. Ammonia is turned into the safer urea, and alcohol is changed to acetaldehyde and then to carbon dioxide and water, so that we do not stay drunk even if we have consumed slightly more than is good for us. But there is a limit to the amount of alcohol the liver can cope with and as we shall see, too much can be harmful to its various complex functions.

27

The kidneys

The two kidneys lie high in the abdomen against the inner back wall, and just on either side of the spine. Large arteries run to them and large veins emerge from them, and these connect with the main, central artery and vein of the body. In this way, all circulating blood passes through the kidneys about once every four or five minutes and without kidneys we would die in a few days. Essentially, they can be regarded as filters which selectively remove from the blood those substances which are either harmful to the body, or which are present in the blood-stream in excess quantity. So the kidneys have a regulating as well as an excretory function and this they perform very efficiently. We can manage perfectly well on one kidney only and could get by, if necessary, with about half of the remaining kidney non-functional.

From each kidney, a narrow tube called the ureter runs downward and into the rear lower part of the urinary bladder. This is an extensible, muscular-walled bag which can stretch and enlarge as it fills with urine. After a time the bladder refuses to expand further and we have to empty it voluntarily. If this is not done, the bladder will eventually release the controlling 'sphincters' and contract involuntarily. The tube from the bladder to the outside is called the urethra and in the male the part of the urethra nearest the bladder is surrounded by the prostate gland.

The reproductive organs

In the male these are closely associated with the urinary system, the same tube, the urethra, serving as a channel for both semen and urine. Sperms develop in the testicles which hang in the scrotum and pass up by way of a tube, on either side, called the *vas deferens* to two little bags called the seminal vesicles. These lie behind the bladder and open into the prostate gland and from there into the urethra. The seminal vesicles secrete a thick nutrient fluid and the sperms mix with this secretion to form the seminal fluid which is stored in the vesicles until rising pressure requires its release.

The urethra runs along the inside of the penis surrounded by three columns of spongy 'erectile' tissue which, when flooded with blood become enlarged and firm. During sexual excitement, the arteries supplying the penis with blood dilate and a fair quantity of blood enters under pressure. This causes the veins which drain the penis to be compressed so that the blood cannot readily get out. When the arteries constrict, more blood leaves than enters and the erection is lost. The control of the penile arteries is much influenced by their owner's state of mind and it is for this reason that most cases of impotence are of psychological rather than of organic origin. During orgasm, the seminal vesicles contract and expel the seminal fluid.

In women, the ovaries lie, one on each side of the pelvis and are joined to the womb by the uterine tubes. The older name for these is the 'fallopian' tubes. Each month, about the middle of the menstrual cycle, one or more tiny eggs (or 'ova') are released from the ovary and carried along the appropriate uterine tube to the uterus. If an ovum meets some seminal fluid, a spermatozoon may penetrate and fertilise it and a pregnancy will result. The fertilised ovum embeds itself in the inner wall of the uterus, forms a placenta and goes on dividing to form an embryo. After 40 weeks the baby is ready to be born.

Over-view

We have been concerned to give you the minimum outline of body structure and function so that you will be able to understand the subsequent chapters. You have seen how the brain is the really essential organ – the seat of the mind and emotions and the ultimate centre of all pleasure and satisfaction. You have also seen that to a large extent, the rest of the body serves as a kind of administrative back-up and transportation vehicle for the brain. It processes and supplies fuel and oxygen so that the brain can continue to function efficiently and be carried where it wishes.

It would be a mistake, however, to leave you with the impression that the mind is an entity totally separated from

29

the body and dissociated from it. Far from it. The mind and the body are so closely inter-related that it is impossible for any major alteration to occur in one without the other being affected. We are all of us acutely aware of our bodies and of their shapes and shortcomings, but we should never make the mistake of thinking that our bodies are more important than our minds. The brain, which is the fount and origin of the mind, is the central and fundamentally important part of us. Although this book will be largely dedicated to the body and the means of ensuring that it does its job properly, it must also be concerned with maintaining the health of the brain and the proper happiness, satisfaction and comfort of the mind.

2 How to assess your health

Now that you know something of how the body works, you will find it easier to make an intelligent assessment of your health and to judge when professional advice is required to ensure you have a healthy lifestyle. Symptoms and signs (symptoms are subjective, signs objective) are important, and some idea of their significance is essential. We shall deal with some symptom groups in this chapter, laying major emphasis on symptoms relating to heart trouble. But you may well be entirely free of specific and obvious symptoms or signs, such as pain, undue breathlessness, weakness, stiffness, and so on. In that case the general state of your health is determined by making an assessment of your overall performance. You must try to do this in both the physical and the mental spheres as only then can you have a healthy lifestyle.

Assessing physical status

Physical performance is essentially a matter of exercise tolerance, and this varies over wide limits. It is important for you to do two things:

(1) become so familiar with the concept of exercise tolerance that you are regularly aware of your own and that of others,

(2) be able to place yourself accurately in the exercise tolerance hierarchy.

This is a scale at the top end of which are the international athletes and at the bottom those who are bedridden. The scale is calibrated in terms of the distance which you can travel, at a brisk pace, before severe breathlessness, or other effects, bring you to a halt. Unfortunately, most of us are somewhere near the bottom of the scale and that, therefore, is where we need to take a closer look.

When doctors are taking a history and trying to determine the severity of a heart or respiratory condition in a patient, they use exercise tolerance as the most sensitive guide because it is a parameter which can be quantified. No such medical assessment would be complete without attempting to gain a rough idea of how far the patient can go before the body 'puts on the brakes'. A patient with angina (a symptom caused by inadequate blood supply to the heart muscle) may be able to walk 100 metres before being stopped by pain. Another may only be able to go 20 metres before the symptom occurs.

If you are a senior executive it is probable that your exercise tolerance will not be at the same level as that of an athlete. If, however, it is because, for instance, you jog regularly then you have already gone a long way to doing yourself a power of good. If you are not even on to the brisk walking scale, then you are heading for trouble, or may already have reached it. A useful rough check of exercise tolerance is your performance on stairs. How do you go up the stairs – one step at a time? Or two or three? Or do you use the stairs at all? When you walk up stairs with a colleague how does your performance compare with his. Can either of you still carry on a conversation while climbing steadily, or are you both so breathless that talking is impossible?

So the first step in assessing your physical status is to try to see where you are on the scale and whether you are sliding down it with increasing age. Note that it is *not* important to try to get as high in the scale as possible. What matters is (a) that you should know where you stand and (b) that your position in the scale should be appropriate to your lifestyle and adequate to maintain health.

Figure 3 — Exercise tolerance levels

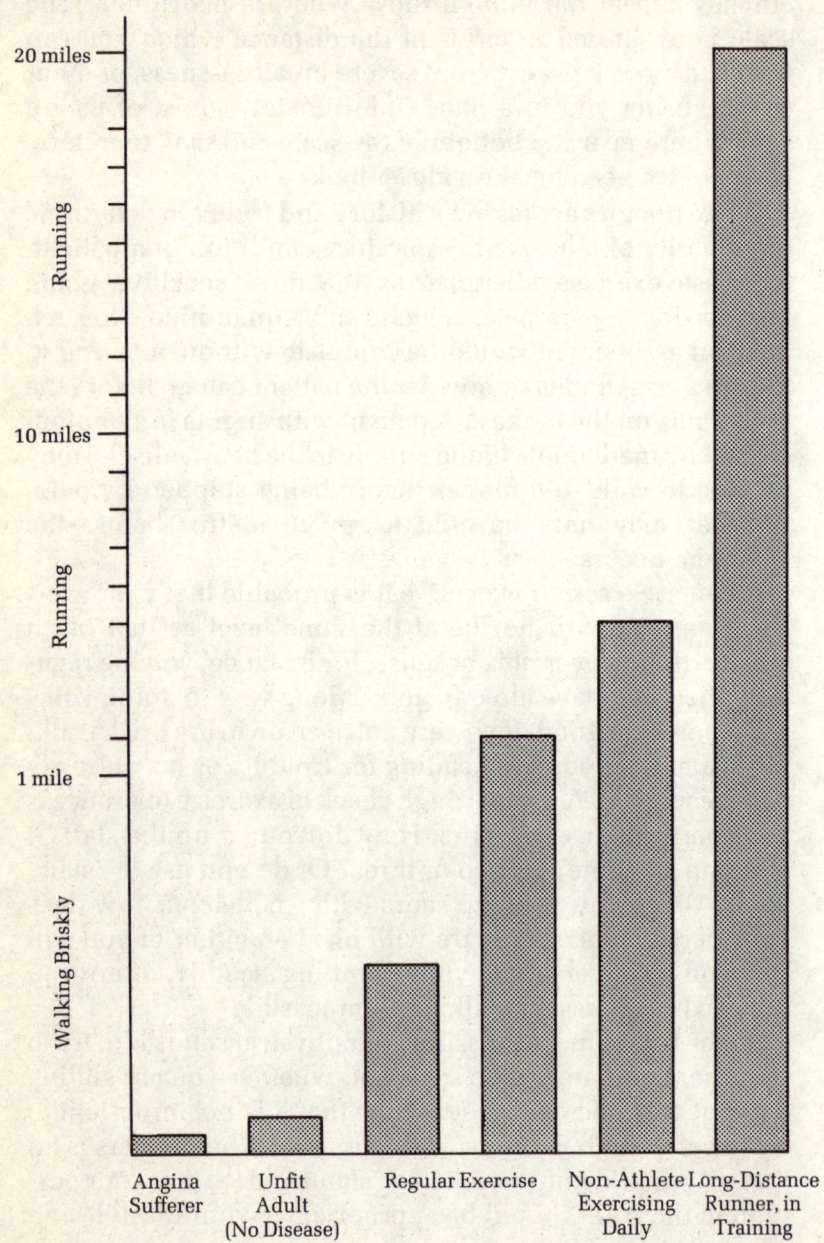

Here are some general guidelines as to what you should be able to do. These refer to a man or woman well into middle age, not particularly concerned with athletic pursuits and not playing physical games regularly. If you feel you should test yourself, please note the following points. Sudden strenuous exertion by the unfit may be dangerous. So discuss the matter with your doctor first, particularly if you are overweight, a heavy smoker, or totally unaccustomed to exercise.

(1) You should be able to walk an indefinite distance, at your own pace – certainly 10 miles.

(2) You should be able to walk at a brisk pace for at least a mile without becoming too breathless.

(3) You should be able to continue after this, at a more normal pace, without difficulty.

(4) You should be able to run up a flight of 20 steps in seven bounds and show no sign of distress.

(5) You should be able, in an emergency, to run 30 metres in well under seven seconds.

No doubt these rather gentle standards will make the young and active smile. While we must be realistic and recognise that patterns of social behaviour have worked against us in the past, we should also recognise that our ability to meet these parameters ought not to be age-related. Obviously, in the real world exercise tolerance *is* related to age, just as the weight tables are. But this is a reflection of the general failure of certain geographic centres of population to resist the temptation of over indulgence. The life insurance weight tables merely show averages, not ideal weight. It is true to a limited extent that muscle bulk and cardio-respiratory efficiency decline with age. Up to the age of about 70, however, these physiological changes are usually minor when compared to the decline in fitness resulting from sedentary living and an unwise diet.

Breathlessness and an increase in the pulse rate are normal responses to exertion and merely indicate that the body is using up oxygen faster than normal rates of respiration and

35

heart beat can supply it. The amount of breathlessness and increased heart rate for a given degree of exertion does, however, vary with the state of fitness. Athletes usually have slow resting pulse rates. Sometimes as slow as 50 per minute compared with the usual 70 to 80. If the heart begins to lose efficiency at, say, 160 beats per minute, the average person may only be able to double the efficient output while the athlete may be able to treble it.

But circulatory efficiency is not just a matter of speeding up the heart. In a trained athlete the heart output, in litres per minute, may rise from the resting value of 5 to an astonishing 35. This seven-fold increase is also due to the greater power and efficiency of heart muscle contraction with each beat so that the stroke volume (the volume of blood pumped per beat) rises.

So do not worry about breathlessness on effort. This is normal and desirable. Everyone should get breathless every day as a matter of deliberate policy, for it is only by so doing that you are likely to improve your exercise tolerance. By walking up the stairs, instead of using the lift you will achieve a better blood supply to all parts of your body. There is also the possibility that by regularly increasing the rate of blood flow you may decrease the rate at which cholesterol is deposited in the walls of your blood vessels.

What you should worry about is getting breathless on minimal effort or on a degree of effort which causes no observable effect on other reasonably healthy people. If this happens then either you are very unfit or you may be suffering from overt organic disease of the heart, blood vessels or lungs.

It should be apparent that the body is wonderfully adaptable to the level of performance required of it. This adaptability is at its peak in youth, but it is a mistake to assume that it is lost altogether later in life. In general, the degree of fitness adjusts itself fairly quickly to our requirement and unfortunately this adjustment works in both directions. So the physically idle executive, unconcerned about bodily welfare, will be just fit enough to make it from bed to table, from table to car and from car to the well-padded chair at his desk. Feedback from the resultant poor levels of performance will ensure that a car, or lift, always awaits his every transportation need and any possibility of improvement in fitness is precluded.

The effective standard rationalisation here is that his time is so precious he simply cannot afford to waste it on walking. There may be something in this and walking may well cost him a pound a step, but can the benefits of ongoing good health be equated with pounds and pence?

Formal exercise tolerance tests are an important part of the specialist medical assessment of your heart. Should you fall into the hands of a cardiologist, the chances are that you will end up on a treadmill, pounding along on one spot, while a technician urges you to greater efforts and a leash of wires connects you to an electrocardiogram. The study of the ECG taken while you are exercising can tell the physician much more than the ECG taken at rest. If you have been having chest pain which cannot be attributed to less alarming causes, this kind of investigation can often give diagnostically useful or reassuring information.

Symptoms

Chest pain

This is one of the most worrying symptoms a man can experience. I say 'man' because chest pain is essentially a male concern. Women, at least until after the menopause, enjoy a remarkable measure of protection from coronary artery disease. So female executives have fewer worries on this score.

Chest pain, to the average middle-aged man, is no joke. If ever you see a prosperous-looking gentleman pause in his hasty transit of the concourse at Waterloo Station and gaze with distracted thoughtfulness at the clock, the chances are that he is fixed in agonising doubt as to whether his chest pain is more indigestion or something worse. Perhaps some clarification would help.

Many conditions cause chest pain and the great majority of

them are not particularly serious. Most chest pains do *not* signify heart trouble. Causes include heartburn, wind, hunger, pleurisy and bronchitis to mention but a few. The two which cause the most concern are angina pectoris and the pain of a coronary thrombosis, but these are by no means the commonest cause of chest pain.

Pain which is constantly, or frequently, present unrelated to exertion, emotion or stress and which in no way interferes with activity is unlikely to be due to a heart problem.

Angina is due to an insufficient blood supply reaching the heart so that the body is capable of a certain amount of exertion without pain. Beyond a certain degree of exertion the pain begins, but on resting it is relieved. The pain of angina pectoris is usually felt just behind the breast-bone and may be no more than a vague aching sensation. More often it is fairly severe and may rapidly develop into terror accompanied by a conviction of impending death. The pain may extend to the left shoulder and run down the inside of the left arm as far as the fingers. Alternatively it may pass through to the back of the chest and up into the neck as far as the jaw. It is worsened when the exertion follows a meal and is exaggerated in cold weather.

The features of angina are usually so constant for any particular individual that any change in the pattern – increased intensity, longer duration, lesser stimulus – must be viewed with gravity, for these indicate an increased probability of major trouble. They are also so characteristic that doctors can reach a high degree of certainty as to the diagnosis, on the basis of the history alone. It must, therefore, be emphasised that if you are having chest pain regularly, you should certainly see your doctor. This is particularly urgent if the pain is brought on by exertion. If the pain does occur cancel your meeting – however urgent it is – and go straight to your doctor.

There are snags in dismissing chest pain as mere 'indigestion'. If you look at the matter calmly and logically you will probably be able to arrive at the true cause. Do remember that angina is sometimes accompanied by abdominal discomfort and a 'bloated' feeling and that it may even be relieved by belching. So look at the whole picture, record it, analyse it, and try to provide your doctor with all the data he needs to come to an accurate conclusion.

Coronary thrombosis, sometimes called 'myocardial infarction' need hardly be described for if it happens you are unlikely to be in a fit state to ask yourself questions. Why 'myocardial infarction'? 'Myo-' means 'muscle', '-cardial' means 'of the heart' and 'infarction' is the state when the vital blood supply to something has been cut off. A coronary thrombosis is a blockage of a coronary artery branch by the formation of blood clot in the lining of the artery, causing infarction of part of the heart muscle. This part dies and, if you survive, heals by scar tissue thereby weakening the power of contraction of that part of the heart. The infarction may involve the full thickness of the wall of the heart, or only a part of it.

The pain is similar to that of angina, but usually much more severe and lasting much longer. Very occasionally, a coronary can be painless and will be shown up by ECG and other tests.

Breathlessness

Once again there are many causes and you should look out for some obvious change in the pattern of breathlessness, or new associated symptoms. You should certainly be well aware of how breathless you get on a given amount of exertion. If you are not, you are either incredibly fit, or so under-exercised that you are probably dangerously unfit. The latter is by far the more likely. Be particularly concerned about breathlessness which starts suddenly.

Breathlessness may be caused, amongst other things, by general unfitness, smoking, obesity, heart disorder, respiratory infection or asthma.

Headache

Just as people with chest pain worry about the state of their coronary arteries, so people with headache worry about brain tumours. Such worry is rarely justified, for among all persistent headache sufferers only a tiny proportion have a tumour. Some pain can be caused by eye strain – reading too many reports in poor light. Persistent headache can be divided into three main groups. The largest group – over three-quarters of the total – contains the tension headaches. These are the stress-related headaches, so common nowadays, which arise as a result of bodily reflection of the state of the sufferer's mind.

Civilised mores demand that we should not respond to our difficulties by screaming, or kicking the cat. Instead, we keep various muscle groups in a state of constant tension, sometimes for hours on end. The selected muscles vary from person to person, but are commonly those around the eyes and in the forehead or at the back of the neck and in the scalp. Some people literally do cause us a pain the neck – your boss or your secretary could be difficult to deal with. Sustained muscle contraction causes pain and this unconscious abuse of muscle is the commonest cause of headache. Recognition of the cause followed by deliberate relaxation will usually bring relief.

The next largest headache group contains the migraines – a term often used incorrectly. True migraine is caused by transient spasm of one or more of the arteries supplying the brain with blood. The effects, during the stage of spasm, can give a remarkable preview of what it is like to suffer neurological disturbance during a stroke. Thus, you can lose half your field of vision for 20 minutes, experience sensory loss in the face or other parts of the body, possibly even have half your body partly paralysed – all with full recovery within half an hour. The blood vessel spasm is a fairly reliable 'fail-safe' mechanism, in that the muscles in the vessels concerned need blood to go on contracting. The next stage, therefore, is one of wide dilation and this is what causes the headache, or so most doctors believe. Symptomatically, the first stage can occur without the second or the second without the first. So now you know whether or not that life-long 'migraine' really is.

The third, quite tiny group contains the large collection of different organic conditions which can cause headache. This group certainly covers brain tumours, but it also contains a great many other conditions – meningitis; high blood pressure; toxic effects of alcohol, carbon monoxide, lead, arsenic; sinusitis; middle ear infections; previous head injury; and so on.

Organic brain disease, such as tumour or abscess, is unlikely to cause headache without some other effects and because of the comprehensive control effected by the brain, these may involve any function of the body. Especially likely to be affected by brain tumour are the visual fields and control of eye movements. So double vision of sudden onset *may* mean trouble. It may also mean one of half a dozen other much less serious problems. Loss of visual field is always an indication that something major is going on, either in the brain or in the eyes themselves. Your fields should extent out sideways to about 80 degrees from straight ahead, but are limited above, below and inwards by the shape of your face. If you want to test them, cover one eye at a time and fix your gaze firmly on a point straight ahead of you while assessing how far you can see to the sides.

Other symptoms and signs

There is no end to these, so only a brief selection, with an outline of their significance, is possible. Never ignore symptoms but consider each carefully and calmly, and act sensibly. Here are some general pointers and a few important specific recommendations.

Pain, the commonest symptom, is a warning that some abnormal process is going on. Most pain denotes fairly trivial upset and common experience shows what may be safely disregarded or treated with simple analgesics such as paracetamol. Note the duration, however. Chronic, persistent, or frequently recurring pain, wherever it may be, should certainly be investigated. New pains, with no obvious cause, and pains in areas not previously affected should, unless transient, also be reported to your doctor.

Cough is so common that it is often disregarded. Here again persistence and change especially may indicate serious trouble. One of the many snags of smoking is that this provides you with an explanation for your chronic cough so that you may feel you need look no further to account for it. Most times you will be right, but the time you are wrong is apt to be the last one. Smokers have to be critically sensitive to any alteration in the character of the cough, and to the development of additional symptoms such as chest pain.

Blood in the urine, vomited blood or altered blood (stuff like dark coffee grounds), coughed-up blood, or tarry blackening of the stools (which indicates that there has been bleeding into the upper part of the gut) should always be investigated without delay. If the blood in the stools remains red this usually indicates it comes from piles, but may arise from more serious trouble in the rectum. Much of such bleeding is of fairly innocent origin, but it could be dangerous to make assumptions.

If you are a middle aged executive – or beyond – any obvious change in your bowel habit, especially unexplained con-

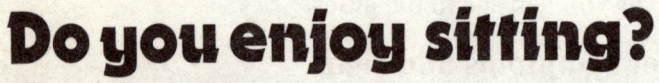
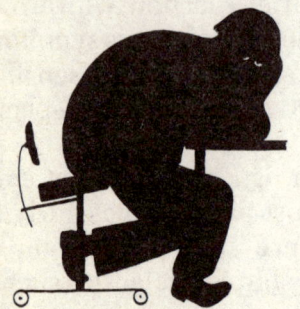

stipation or a continuing alteration in the configuration of the stools, could indicate trouble in the intestine.

Symptoms and signs related to the urinary system are common. Women get burning on urinating, frequency, stress incontinence. Men get these, too, but also may have major problems in emptying the bladder because of enlargement of the prostate, so that they constantly have the desire to urinate. The volume and force of the urine stream is the best layman's guide to the state of the prostate. It is all right to get up once or twice a night, but more often implies either insomnia, excessive fluid intake or prostate trouble.

Frequency of urination, with the production of large volumes of urine and a corresponding thirst suggests diabetes. If you are losing weight and having focusing problems, the probability rises to 90 per cent. If, in addition, your urine splashes dry white, the diagnosis is certain.

Assessing mental effectiveness

This is more difficult, mainly because you are using the tool to measure itself. You will, therefore, have to be very detached and honest in your judgement and take special note of objective criteria. You are likely to try to rationalise away any decline in those essential powers which are central to your whole value as an executive. To do so may be a feature of the problem. Such rationalisation may be good for your *amour propre*, but it is not going to have any bearing on how others see and assess you. That is what really matters and this is a case where, if there is a problem, only 'know thyself' can help.

Some aspects of apparent mental deterioration do increase with age, the most striking being the power of the memory. Many senior executives suffer from *'La maladie des petits morceaux du papier'* and compensate excellently, vying with their peers in the skill with which they conceal the matter. But there are other features which should be noted because some of them are indications of cerebral underfunctioning which may be remediable.

The most frequent of the several causes of this kind of problem is inadequacy of blood supply to the brain, usually from a general atherosclerosis (see Glossary) of the blood vessels supplying the brain and their small branches within the brain. But sometimes the main reason for the poor blood supply lies in one or more of the four major arteries taking blood up to the head – the carotids and the vertebrals. These may become critically narrowed by disease, and surgery can help. However, this is not an easy procedure, nor one casually adopted by any doctor. Whilst this is certainly not the commonest cause of under-perfusion of the brain, when it is, treatment can sometimes make a world of difference to the person concerned.

Clearly, mental effectiveness is going to vary from day to day. All sorts of subtle factors, many of them external, will see to that. Judged over a period it should, however, be possible to determine whether you show an appreciable change in any of the following characteristics:

(1) ability to cope with everyday matters;

(2) speed with which new ideas are grasped;

(3) characteristic mood;

(4) performance in skilled activities requiring good coordination;

(5) neatness of dress and concern about appearance;

(6) consideration for the feelings of others.

Note that in all these, it is a *change* that is significant. If you decide that there has been a major change you should seek medical advice to see whether anything can be done. In addition to arterial problems, other general disorders can affect the efficiency of cerebral function, and many of these are now treatable. A thorough check-up could be the best investment of your life. Most of you as executives will doubtless have examinations carried out by the company's doctor; if these are not done frequently then go to your own doctor.

3 Stress

The stereotype idea of the modern executive is that he is living and working under constant high level stress. Whether or not you agree with this depends largely on your personality type. It also depends on other factors like your general level of competence in dealing with both your business and personal problems. If you feel constantly under stress, it may be difficult to acknowledge that other people exposed to similar stressors may be less affected by them.

Everyone understands what is meant by a stressful situation, for example having your judgement questioned, sitting an important examination, being angry, overworked or frustrated. But to the physiologist, the word 'stress' has a wider meaning. He is interested in the changes that occur in the body as a result of stress. He is also aware that a much wider range of influences can operate to bring about these changes, than we perhaps appreciate.

The man who first wrote about the subject in detail, Hans Selye (he published *Stress* in 1950, and *The Stress of Life* in 1956) is said to have had a language problem and to have picked the wrong term. In engineering 'stress' is the force acting on something to change its dimensions, while 'strain' is the distortion or change caused by the stress. Formerly, the word 'strain' was widely used, much as we use the word 'stress' today for example 'He is under a great strain. . .', and it is suggested that what Selye actually meant was 'strain'.

In fact, Selye's usage was scientifically correct, and it was the general public who were wrong. However, because the correct word was unusual in this context, it quickly caught on and has remained in common usage.

The stressors

Medical men define stress as that range of factors which cause a quite definite and specific set of bodily responses. These factors include overwork; prolonged strong emotion such as anger, jealousy or shame; regular frustration in daily life or employment; persistent loss of sleep; death of a spouse; divorce; and business failure.

In addition, stress also includes actual physical injury, pain, major illness, haemorrhage, severe infection, exposure to cold, and decreased oxygen supply. The thing that all these 'stressors' have in common is that they produce a characteristic response in the form of secretion into the blood of two powerful biochemical substances called hormones. A hormone is a chemical released by one tissue which travels by the blood to a target tissue where it causes a particular response.

Following stress, the initial hormonal response comes from the central hormone controlling gland, the pituitary. This is situated on the underside of the brain and is in close functional connection with it. Pituitary action is very much concerned with, and responsive to, information received by the brain. The result is the production of a range of hormones exerting control over the other endocrine glands of the body. The most important of these, in the context of stress, are the adrenal glands – two small cap-shaped organs sitting on top of the kidneys. Hormones produced by the pituitary result in secondary secretion from the adrenals and these secretions, which flood out into the blood, are cortisol and adrenaline. Cortisol is the natural cortico-steroid of the body and is, of course, widely used as a therapeutic agent.

Now these hormones are produced for a purpose which, in the short term, is advantageous. The well-known beneficial effect of 'stage-fright' on the performance of actors or musicians, is a stress-related phenomenon caused by cortisol and

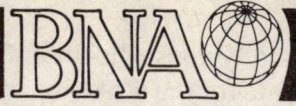

BNA

British Nursing Association

HOW CAN BNA RELIEVE YOUR STRESS?

We recognise that your domestic life, if not running smoothly, will have an effect on you and your performance at work. Ill health in the family, a sick child, or a frail parent will cause you anxiety and concern.

How can BNA help?

By providing a trained nurse, auxiliary or carer in your own home for as long or short a time as you need – visits or on a long term basis. We have over 35,000 health care professionals registered with us, and that includes

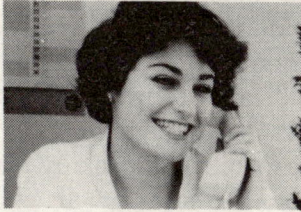

WE ARE ONLY A PHONE CALL AWAY

nannies, health visitors, midwives and occupational health nurses.

BNA has been established for nearly 40 years and is now the largest agency in the UK, providing a nationwide service from over 90 branches from the North of England to Torquay in Devon.

Each BNA branch provides a 24-hour, 7 day week service to ensure that the standard of health care required by you is provided. All our branches are run by caring qualified nurses who are trained to meet your requirements, and every BNA nurse has had their qualifications and references checked – we pride ourselves on being professionals.

If you are responsible for recruiting medical personnel for your company, remember that BNA has many nurses looking for their next permanent position.

Why not contact your local branch to discuss the ways in which BNA can help you?

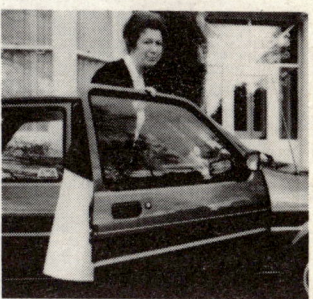

CARE IN YOUR OWN HOME

Let us take the stress away from you!

Find us in Yellow Pages or contact our Head Office at:
North Place, 82 Great North Road, Hatfield, Herts AL9 5BL. 07072 63544

A NESTOR–BNA COMPANY

adrenaline. Biologically these hormonal responses are an attempt to compensate for the stress, or to correct its adverse effects, and are quite essential for a normal, healthy life.

How do they work? Cortisol stimulates catabolism of protein and fat. Catabolism is the breaking-down process whereby energy is liberated for use in work. During this process large biochemical molecules are reduced to simpler substances useful for fuel. Cortisol hastens the conversion of protein products to glucose, the natural fuel of the body. It also ensures that this fuel is made available only to those parts of the body which need it most in the stressful circumstances, notably the brain and the muscles. It also acts on fats, prompting their break down to glycerol and fatty acids, both of which can provide fuels. Note that cortisol increases the levels of fats in the blood.

Adrenaline increases the heart rate and the strength of the heart muscle contraction, reduces fatigue in muscles and shunts blood from the digestive system to the main muscles by causing the blood vessels of the former to close down and those of the latter to open up. It also increases the air intake of the lungs and prompts the release of glucose from the liver. Finally, you should note particularly that adrenaline increases the coagulability of the blood. You may think this is a good thing and for wounds and cuts it may be so. But if we consider clotting actually occurring within the blood vessels – the phenomenon known as 'thrombosis' – you will appreciate that it can have disadvantages.

You will need little other information further to demonstrate that these are powerful and important effects. An animal whose adrenal glands are removed has no source of cortisol or adrenaline and will die if exposed to severe stress. A similar situation arises quite commonly in medical practice. Corticosteroid drugs are invaluable in certain carefully defined circumstances and can often save lives. When treatment with steroids is unavoidable, the doctor prescribes them in the knowledge that the presence of high steroid levels in the blood temporarily knocks out the natural production of cortisol from the adrenals. The administered steroids take over and the normal power to respond to stress may be abolished. So doctors are careful to ensure that patients on steroid treatment carry a card or other indication that steroids are being taken. In the event of a serious accident, anaesthetic or other stress, a large dose of steroids can then be given to see the patient safely over the emergency.

The role of anxiety

No one is entirely clear how the stressors actually lead to the hormonal response. It is generally believed that the signal to the appropriate part of the brain (the bit called the 'hypothalamus', situated just above the stalk of the pituitary) arises automatically when the individual becomes anxious. There is a good deal of evidence for this and the point is important, because anxiety can arise in all sorts of ways, not all of them reasonable or necessary.

In more primitive times, anxiety was largely linked with danger and the stress response provided energy, thus enabling the threatened individual to respond more effectively by fight or flight. The same kind of response also occurs in severe anxiety even if it is the result of some psychiatric disorder, for example agoraphobia, and the sufferer will experience all the physical effects of terror – fast-beating heart, rapid breathing, sweating, tremor, and so on.

A number of studies done on military personnel under battle conditions, have shown a close correlation between the levels of anxiety and the blood cortisol levels. The officers and NCOs who had the greatest personal responsibility showed the highest steroid responses. The same kind of thing has been found in servicemen undergoing arduous training. The cortisol levels rose when new tasks and new equipment were introduced and fell again when these were mastered.

Other cortisol effects

We have not finished with the effects of this remarkable hormone. Large amounts of cortisol interfere severely with inflammation. This is one of the body's most important protective mechanisms against infection and is essential in the process of healing. It has been repeatedly demonstrated in clinical practice that high blood steroid levels allow severe infection to go unchecked, cause dormant infections, such as TB, to flare up and gastric and duodenal ulcers to recur and often to bleed.

Cortisol is a powerful inhibitor of the immune system. Steroids are used routinely to induce a temporary acquired immune deficiency state to prevent the rejection of grafted organs such as kidneys and hearts. It would, of course, be an exaggeration to suggest that stress can cause AIDS. It is no exaggeration, however, to point out that immune deficiency is a relative thing. Susceptibility to many illnesses is undoubtedly brought about through stress-induced cortisol interference with the immune system.

Individuals also vary in the system of the body most sensitive to the stress response. In many the blood pressure and the arteries are affected, but some people show a relatively greater effect on the digestive system, the skin, the kidneys, and so on. Stress may also cause loss of appetite, diarrhoea, sweating, blushing, a rapidly recurring desire to pass urine, or may result in headache. These are all individual variations and indicate the manner in which persistent and unrelieved stress may be expected to affect the individual if stress-related disease arises. Some people will get high blood pressure and heart disease, some will develop skin diseases, like acne rosacea (which could be noticeably more common in our female executives rather than the males), some will get colitis or duodenal ulcers. The direction in which stress acts seems to be closely tied up with personality type and it would be sensible to try to become familiar with the way in which stress affects you, so that you can readily recognise it and perhaps do something about it.

Personality types

Interestingly, studies have shown that different people react to stress by quite wide variations in the extent of the bio-chemical response. Students sitting important oral examina-tions were checked for heart-rate, blood pressure and levels of blood cortisols. All showed a rise during the stress of the examination, but some reacted much more markedly than others and it was found possible to relate the strength of the response to the physical type. As a general rule, burly, athle-tic subjects showed significantly lower levels of cortisol than those of slim build. There is now a great deal of evidence to suggest that the anxious, competitive, driving type of person (the type 'A' personality) is much more prone to diseases such as high blood pressure and coronary thrombosis than the type 'B' person (see following section). All the indica-tions are that a major factor in bringing about this effect is that they are constantly being exposed to stress situations of this kind.

Let us look a little further into this question of the relation-ship of personality to stress-induced illness.

Type 'A' and type 'B' personalities

This section must relate mainly to male readers as there is very little clinical data available regarding women and their reactions to stress.

The type 'A' man is always worrying about time. He has a constant feeling of urgency, works at high speed and always tries to cram as much as possible into the available time. He walks fast, may drive dangerously, and talks impatiently, often interrupting others. To quote one of the original authors of the concept '. . . he is aggressively involved in a chronic, incessant struggle to achieve more and more in less and less time. . .'.

The type 'B' man is very laid-back and has a calm, relaxed outlook on life and a knack of rolling with the punch. He may get just as much work done as his noisy, thrusting colleague, but to watch him you would hardly guess it. In some cases, he may actually get much less work done and his relaxed calm may just be a front for plain laziness.

The first point to make about the comparison between these two groups is that the evidence is purely statistical, and you have to take into account considerable numbers of people before trends can be securely demonstrated. You cannot argue that since type 'A' is a driving, high-pressure, ruthless, competitive pirate he will necessarily succumb to a coronary thrombosis before he is forty-five. However, if you take a number of 'A's and see what happens to them, facts begin to emerge. Although the evidence gives proof of trends only, there is plenty of it. In one trial of over 3,000 men, followed up for eight years, it was found that the type 'A' group had twice as many heart attacks as the type 'B'.

One of the snags is that, whereas some individuals can very readily be put into their type categories, many are hard to classify and could fall into either group. Some research has been devoted to refining this classification and one of the promising and important things to come out of this is the significance of repressed aggression.

Hostility

Studies have shown that the feature of the type 'A' personality most likely to be associated with coronary artery disease is hostility. It is clear that those whose competitiveness is demonstrated by powerful aggression and unconcern for the rights of others are particularly susceptible. Today hostility ratings can easily be determined using routine psychological tests.

The best known and most widely used of these tests is the 'Minnesota Multiphasic Personality Inventory'. The subject has to tick 'true' or 'false' to over 500 statements and the computer analysis of the responses produces a remarkably detailed statement of the personality of the subject. The MMPI can quickly identify, *inter alia*, people with high hostility ratings. When this group of people were followed up, it was found that their death rate from coronary thrombosis and related diseases was six times as high as those with low hostility ratings.

Of course aggression is a self-perpetuating phenomenon, leading to alienation and isolation. This is a major stress factor. Often, the lack of concern for others arises from the conviction that if you do not protect your rear, your competitors will take immediate advantage. To some, aggression is the only logical response and, inevitably, others retaliate. Anxiety and a sense of insecurity result.

Fear of personal disadvantage and constant distrust of others, force the unfortunate victim into a state of constant watchfulness, continually ready for fight or flight. The natural physiological response is high blood levels of cortisol and adrenaline – and you know what these do.

Open hostility is generally acknowledged to be dangerous. That people get apoplexy from high blood pressure in the course of excessive anger is notorious. We now also know that habitual, repressed hostility is the real risk factor. A study at Duke University, North Carolina, showed that the stress effects of bottling up strong hostility were so serious that this factor alone could account for the higher levels of serious arterial disease in type 'A' people.

The theory has still to receive general acceptance, but if it is correct there may be much to learn from it. Many of the best qualities of the type 'A' man may after all be harmless, so long as aggression is adequately controlled and properly directed. Perhaps you should take a detached look at your relationships with others and see how aggression is generated and how it can be dispersed. If you can come to accept that the dangers of aggressive selfishness outweigh the satisfaction of 'scoring' over others, perhaps some unpleasant consequences can be avoided.

Stress and the heart

As already mentioned, the increase in the amount of circulating cortisol during stress, results in fatty acids being mobilised from the fat stores of the body and released into the blood circulation. These fats pass to the liver where they are converted to cholesterol and this, in turn, is released into the bloodstream. So stress causes a rise in the amount of cholesterol in the blood which is bad news for the blood vessels and heart. However, cholesterol is not the only stress-produced substance which can harm the heart, adrenaline too has a very sensitive and immediate effect on raising the blood pressure. As you will read in the next chapter, raised blood pressure is one of the main risk factors leading to atherosclerosis. If severe, this is a disaster, not only for the heart but for every other organ in the body supplied by affected arteries and particularly the brain.

Recognising anxiety

Signs of the 'fright, fight or flight' reaction vary a good deal from one person to another and the common indications such as trembling, tense muscles, dry mouth, sweating, pounding of the heart and so on, need not all necessarily occur. Nevertheless, it is important for you to be able to recognise the particular way in which you respond physically to anxiety, so that you can do something (such as formal relaxation exercises) to minimise the effects. People who respond to stress are seldom aware of the sort of situation that produces it. So a careful analysis of the physical symptoms caused can be of great value.

When people are under stress, their bodies tend to take up a quite characteristic position and those of us with this problem must learn to recognise it at once. Many of the following signs may be observed in a person under stress. The jaw is clenched and the muscles of the face are contracted; the forehead is wrinkled and the eyes wide open, or sometimes, tightly screwed up; the head is pushed forward and the shoulders are held high up towards the ears; the fists are tightly clenched and the arms are tightly folded and pressed firmly against the body which is bent forward a little and held very stiffly. If the person is sitting, the legs are usually crossed tightly and the upper foot often points upwards and if standing, there is a tendency to restless walking about.

Maintaining such a posture actually increases stress, as

you will find if you try it and a vicious cycle is set up which leads to exhaustion. So obviously, the thing to do is to learn to relax. Some people find it relatively easy to do this without help, but many require assistance.

Stress events and illness

It will now come as no surprise to you to learn that doctors have long recognised that there is a strong correlation between stressful events in life and the subsequent development of illness. Many of these associations are commonplace. For instance shingles, which is caused by the flare-up of viruses which have lain dormant in the nervous system since that childhood attack of chickenpox, are the result of a reduction in immune capacity. This, in turn, is often the demonstrable result of external stress. An attack of shingles often follows events such as bereavement, accident or another major illness.

Interestingly, the events which are followed by a breakdown in health, do not seem always to be unpleasant. Rather, they seem to be events which call for a major change, or readjustment, of the life pattern of the person concerned. A good many research studies have shown that major changes are commonly followed by severe illness. To test this idea, scales were produced which give a score for events thought to be significant. By the use of these scales attempts have been made to predict illness in large groups of people, with remarkable success.

One of the best known was that of Holmes and Rahe who headed their scale with a figure of 100 for the death of a spouse, gave 73 for divorce, 65 for marital separation, and so on down to 11 for a minor violation of the law. When this scale was used they found, for instance, that someone scoring a total of 300 or more had a 90 per cent chance of suffering a decline in health. The most dangerous circumstance seems to be combinations of these events occurring within a short period. Later studies supported the claim and drew particular attention to the relationship between such changes and coronary heart disease. Attempted suicide also correlated closely with many such stress trigger events.

You may think that all this is no more than plain common sense, but there are plenty of people around who live as if they are quite unaware of the potential danger. Obviously, many of these events are entirely outside our control, but this by no means applies to all and you often have choice in determining their timing. In any event, being aware of the particular effect that stress has upon you and the times at which you are especially vulnerable does, if you are sensible and informed, provide the possibility of doing something to minimise the effects. 'Know thyself' said the Greek philosopher Thales and that principle is as true today as it was 2,700 years ago.

4 High blood pressure and heart disease

Now comes the crux of the matter. Almost all the other subjects already covered have a bearing on the central question of the health of the heart and blood vessels. If this book can succeed in raising your awareness of the importance of this fact, it will have achieved much. The fact that a book on executive health care lays so much emphasis on heart disease must not be taken to imply that executives, as a group, have a greater risk than others of developing coronary artery disease. In fact, this is not so. Knowledge, intelligence and the capacity to allow reason to rule the inclinations – so that knowledge is intelligently applied in altering lifestyle patterns – are the only hope of reversing this modern plague. It is, therefore, encouraging to be able to report that enlightenment has already had a notable impact on the statistics. There is also clear evidence that the greater part of this reduction has occurred in those groups who are accustomed to learn, think and act accordingly.

To the executive, as to everyone else, the matter is vital – and for once, the much-abused word 'vital' is applied literally. The DHSS annual report for 1985 shows that no less than 163,104 people died from coronary artery disease in England and Wales. That figure accounts for 28 per cent of all deaths, strikingly ahead of all other causes. The second commonest cause of death, at 12 per cent, was 'stroke' due to disease of blood vessels supplying the brain. Another 9 per cent were due to various other conditions involving the

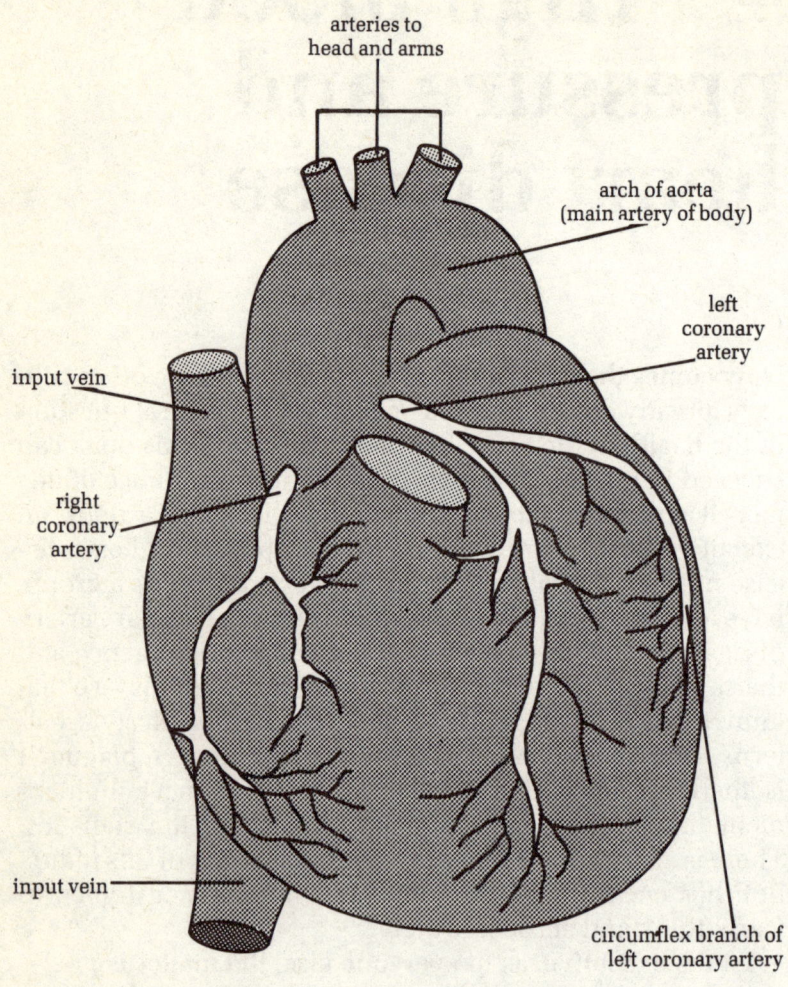

Figure 4 — Coronary arteries arising from the Aorta

arteries. Together, these made up about 287,000 deaths, all of them attributable to an unhealthy state of the arteries in people like us.

So nearly half of all those dying each year do so because their arteries are unable to maintain an adequate supply of blood to the heart muscle or to the brain. This inability results from the condition known as atherosclerosis, a lumpiness of the inner lining of the arteries caused by deposits of cholesterol and other materials. Normally, blood will never clot within healthy blood vessels. Conversely, this lack of internal smoothness in the arteries produces the constant risk that blood will clot on top of the lumps.

The abnormal clotting of blood within a blood vessel is called a thrombosis. When such clots occur, the artery concerned can become blocked. Vital blood is unable to get through and the tissue supplied by the artery, whatever it may be, simply dies. If this tissue should be a part of the heart muscle then its death is obviously very serious. Should the artery concerned be a large one, the heart is likely to be stopped. This is what is known as cardiac arrest.

It is not only death we are concerned with, however. The mortality figures quoted also reflect an enormous amount of chronic ill-health, disability and distress. For instance, people who have had non-fatal coronaries may be left with severely injured hearts, capable of only a fraction of the output needed for normal living. In such cases any exertion causes severe cardiac discomfort (angina pectoris) and breathlessness and such a person may have to be confined to a bed or a chair.

Risk factors

The chief risk factors associated with arterial disease of this kind are:

(1) Cigarette smoking. The more smoked, the greater the danger.

(2) High blood pressure. The higher the pressure, the greater the danger.
(3) Blood cholesterol levels. The higher the level, the greater the danger.
(4) Obesity. The greater the weight, the greater the danger.
(5) Stress. Stress factors relate to personality type.
(6) Physical laziness. The greater the amount of regular exertion, the lower the danger.

Let us now look at the relationship between high blood pressure (often called 'hypertension') and disease of the blood vessels and heart.

High blood pressure

Approximately 15 per cent of people in the western world have high blood pressure and most of them are unaware of it. In many with mild hypertension, the condition seems to be harmless and often settles without treatment or amendment of lifestyle. But 10 to 12 per cent of these people, although experiencing no symptoms, suffer a gradual rise in pressure. This increase continues until serious damage has been done to the blood vessels and the organs they supply. The condition is then too far advanced for treatment to be effective.

So it is no good waiting until the hypertension shows itself by its effects on the arteries. The condition has to be looked for. There is no critical level at which high blood pressure suddenly causes arterial disease. Analysis of a mass of clinical data shows that the number of people with coronary artery and other arterial diseases rises steadily with increased blood pressure. All this adds up to the fact that whether you suspect you have hypertension or not, you should have blood pressure checks at least once a year to ensure that all is well.

The causes of high blood pressure

In about 85 per cent of cases of hypertension, even the most refined methods of investigation will fail to find a cause. All we know is that the trouble tends to run in families and that it is commoner in populations with a high salt intake. The other 15 per cent of sufferers have hypertension from a discoverable cause, such as kidney disease, narrowing of the aorta (the main artery of the body), etc.

Once hypertension is well established and has begun to cause damage to the arteries, however, a vicious cycle starts in which progressive loss of elasticity in the arteries leads in turn to raised blood pressure. Obviously, if a pulse of pressure is applied to a tube the rise will depend on how easily the tube can 'give' under that pressure. So there is an inseparable relationship between blood pressure and arterial disease, which is just as close as the relationship between arterial disease and heart disease.

Hypertension in the early stages is easily and effectively treated, often without any side-effects whatsoever. Once it is fully established and the damage has been done, treatment is of limited value. The moral is surely clear!

High blood pressure and salt intake

The evidence that salt intake is an important factor in causing hypertension has aroused much controversy and the arguments are still going on. Some points are clear. Doctors have known for a long time, that rigid restriction in salt intake causes a major fall in blood pressure, in people with severe hypertension. This is often adopted as part of their treatment. There is also evidence, although it is less secure, that restriction to about half of the average intake will bring down moderate or mild hypertension, at least in some people. When various communities are compared, it has been found that the higher the salt intake the greater the number of people with high blood pressure. For instance in Belgium and Japan – communities with traditionally high salt intake – government intervention has resulted in a fall in salt intake. This has been followed by a reduction in the prevalence of high blood pressure and mortality from stroke.

Evidence of this kind should be looked at very critically as it is somewhat circumstantial, and factors other than salt restriction may be operating. However, many specialists consider it strong enough to justify advising a reduction in salt consumption. It is pointed out that we eat 10 to 20 times as much salt as is physiologically necessary and that reduction to much lower levels cannot do any harm.

Interestingly, and contrary to expectation, adaptation to a low salt regime is not particularly difficult. Food certainly tastes uninteresting at first, but within two or three weeks the taste-buds adapt and increase their sensitivity to salinity. New subtilities of flavour appear and salty food becomes unpleasant.

The idea is simply to avoid salt in cooking, avoid highly salted foods and add no salt to food at table. This halves the salt intake and it is likely we would all be the better for it.

The causes of atherosclerosis

You may be surprised, and perhaps alarmed, to learn that atherosclerosis starts in childhood. The first thing that happens is that the innermost layer of the artery becomes unnaturally thickened. It can be seen happening quite early in life. When, as often happens in males, there are well localised areas of excessive thickening, it is possible to accurately predict that these areas are where atherosclerosis is going to occur later. This is a sobering thought.

These areas of thickening do not significantly interfere with the flow of blood, but by the time we reach our late twenties and early thirties, a more ominous sign may often be detected. This is the presence, on top of these thickened patches of soft, yellow, raised fatty plaques. These consists mainly of cholesterol and become both more numerous and more prominent as time passes. They commonly occur in the coronary arteries, and are appearing much more often in younger people than was formerly the case.

The actual mechanism by which these dangerous plaques occur is not yet fully understood, but there is considerable evidence to indicate that high blood pressure contributes to their development. It seems likely that undue stretching, turbulence and shear forces, secondary to the high pressure, cause damage to the lining membrane and allow the fats access.

Obviously, the levels of cholesterol in the blood are also important. People with very low blood cholesterol levels simply do not have the material available for the production of atherosclerosis. This is borne out by post-mortem examination of the arteries of people who have always had a very low fat diet. These are completely free from atherosclerosis.

The arteries of cigarette smokers have, of course, received a great deal of attention and post-mortem studies show a close correlation between the degree of atherosclerosis and the number of cigarettes smoked. This subject is dealt with more fully in Chapter 5 but it should be emphasised here that once severe atherosclerosis has developed, there is very little that can be done to reduce it. The moral is clear. Those factors leading to the condition should be eliminated at the earliest possible stage, for example, by actively dissuading young people from starting to smoke.

Angina pectoris

A person with angina can usually remain reasonably comfortable if exertion or strong emotion is avoided, but after a variable amount of physical exertion, or on becoming angry or anxious, the symptom starts. In an early or mild case, a fair amount of exertion may be necessary, but the condition tends to become progressively worse as time passes. Later on the angina may even occur when the person concerned is at rest.

Angina produces a sense of extreme discomfort in the middle of the chest and often in the left arm and neck. It is more like a tight, gripping band than a sharp pain and the feeling in the arm is often one of numbness and weakness. When the angina radiates to the neck, there can be a sense of choking. Most attacks last for two or three minutes and are relieved by rest or control of emotions. Such an attack is often accompanied by a terrifying feeling that death is about to occur.

Ninety per cent of cases of this distressing condition are

caused by atherosclerosis of the coronary arteries. At post-mortem examination at least one of the three main coronary arteries is usually found to be narrowed, by plaques, to about 20 per cent of its normal internal diameter. Often two or three of the main vessels are affected in this way. People with angina often live for a surprisingly long time. About 50 per cent live for ten years or more from the time of onset, but survival depends largely on how many of the coronary arteries are markedly narrowed. Of those in whom all three main vessels are affected, one in ten will die each year.

Coronary thrombosis

When a blood clot builds up on a plaque of atherosclerosis in a coronary artery and causes complete closure of the vessel, the outcome depends on the size of the vessel involved. The location of the symptom is the same as in angina, but now the person feels a choking, bursting or vice-like gripping which, instead of settling after two or three minutes, persists for from half an hour to several hours. One patient in five dies within the first two hours and two patients out of five die within the first month. Of those who survive the first month, about 70 per cent live for five years. In general, mortality varies with age. Younger people survive much better than older people and coronary thrombosis in the elderly carries a high mortality rate.

Sudden death from heart disease

Although severe coronary thrombosis commonly causes sudden death by cutting off the blood supply to the heart muscle, people with coronary atherosclerosis may die suddenly without this having happened. A heart which has been deprived of its proper supply of oxygen and nutrients for a long time, is prone to two main disorders. These may either cause it to stop beating altogether or alter its beat to a rapid, ineffectual twitching called 'ventricular fibrillation'. Both these conditions immediately stop the circulation of blood and death occurs almost at once. (NB There is another kind of fibrillation, involving the upper part of the heart only. This condition, atrial fibrillation, is quite different and does not cause sudden death.)

One of the most potent risk factors in bringing about cardiac arrest is cigarette smoking. The same risk applies, of course, to people who have had coronary thrombosis. For such people to continue to smoke is positively suicidal.

Exercise and blood pressure

Carefully controlled trials have shown that exercise of ten minutes duration, with rests in between, which increases the heart rate to about 120 beats per minute, will cause a drop in the blood pressure of about 25 per cent. This applies equally to people with normal blood pressure and those with hypertension. Such exercise can readily reduce moderately raised blood pressure to normal for periods of four to ten hours afterwards. The exercise may consist of brisk walking or jogging and should be moderate, especially in those with heart disease. It is suggested that if you are over 40, overweight, a smoker, or in any way uncertain as to the safety of this valuable measure in your own case, you should consult your doctor before undertaking it. Mild hypertension can be treated very effectively in this way, without drugs, and the method carries other incidental advantages as indicated in Chapter 7.

Blood cholesterol and coronary heart disease

Cholesterol is carried in the blood in combination with protein, either as 'high density lipo-proteins' or as 'low density lipo-proteins'. It is the latter, the LDLP, that are dangerous. The HDLP are actually protective against atherosclerosis. So when blood cholesterol is discussed, it is LDLP which are referred to.

It is pleasing to be able to report that it has now been proved that reducing very high blood cholesterol (LDLP) levels reduces the chance of coronary heart disease. In 1984, the Journal of the American Medical Association reported the results of a seven-year trial on 3,806 men with high blood cholesterol levels. All the men were put on a diet in which the ratio of polyunsaturated fat to saturated fat was increased (see Chapter 8). In addition, half the men were given a drug, cholestyramine, which lowers blood cholesterol levels, and half an inactive substance. Blood cholesterol was reduced by an average of 14 per cent and these men showed a reduction, in the usual rate of coronary disease, of nearly 20 per cent. In the most co operative, who managed to get their blood cholesterol down by 25 per cent, the level of coronary disease was reduced to less than half the expected amount.

Some very interesting figures were reported at a symposium on lipo-proteins and atherosclerosis in Helsinki in November, 1986. Dr Richard Peto of the Radcliffe Infirmary, Oxford, outlining the combined results of 20 random controlled trials of cholesterol reduction stated that reducing blood cholesterol by 10 per cent, whether by diet or drugs, produced a 16 per cent fall in coronary heart disease after

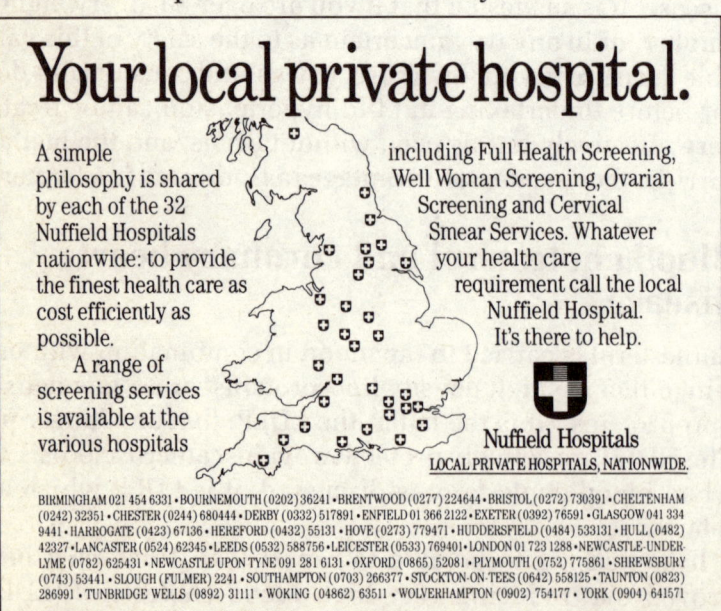

only two years. Dr Peto also referred to studies in rural China where average blood cholesterol levels are roughly half those in the west and where the death rate from coronary heart disease is only 4 per cent of that in Britain.

Please note that these trials do not indicate that lowering the LDLP cholesterol levels will reduce the risk of coronary thrombosis in everyone. The trials have been concerned only with people whose cholesterol levels are higher than average and it is only in such people that the lowering has been proved to be beneficial. Conversley, the trials did not show that lowering cholesterol levels does not reduce the risk of coronary thrombosis. However, since we do not really have any idea of what normal cholesterol levels should be, it is obviously better not to take the risk. Eating polyunsaturated fats (vegetable and fish fats) rather than saturated (animal) fats will lower the levels of cholesterol and this has to be a good thing.

The fish oil controversy

In 1985 a series of articles appeared in the prestigious *New England Journal of Medicine* concerning a suggested inverse association between the consumption of fish and the incidence of coronary artery atherosclerosis. These studies suggested that even a moderate intake of fish oils in the diet may have reduced the incidence of coronary artery disease in both European and North American populations.

In a paper in the *British Medical Journal* in August, 1986, research workers in epidemiology at the National Institute of Environmental Medicine, and the Department of Environmental Hygiene, in Stockholm reported on the findings in a 14 year follow-up of nearly 11,000 subjects in Sweden. This study was most carefully conducted and all subjects who had any record of previous heart trouble were excluded. Differences in age and sex, smoking habits, relative weight, marital status and geographic region were all taken into account. The results were related to a control group who ate little or no fish.

Only death from coronary heart disease was considered in the final analysis. This showed that for every 10 people dying of coronary thrombosis in the low fish consumption group, only seven died in the high consumption group.

Fish oils have to remain liquid at low temperatures and are polyunsaturated fats. The mechanism by which they might reduce the risks of atherosclerosis is unclear although some attractive ideas have been put forward relating them to the function of the blood platelets – the tiny elements important in blood clotting. Substantial data is now available on this subject and is attracting increasing interest, for it offers a possible insight into the ways in which atherosclerosis develops.

That is for the future, however. For now, you should be asking yourself whether you could benefit from these empirical findings. To do so you would probably have to change to an essentially fish protein diet, before you could hope to make a major reduction in your chances of avoiding a coronary. More emphasis on fish can certainly do no harm and there are other good reasons for cutting down on animal proteins – notably the tendency to high calorie intake. So there can be no harm in regularly opting for the Dover sole rather than the Tournedos steak at your favourite restaurant.

Dissolving the clot

Although this book is concerned with prevention rather than cure, you will be interested to learn about something new and exciting in the management of recent coronary thrombosis. Over the years, many attempts have been made to dissolve clots which have formed in diseased blood vessels. The first important drug was the enzyme streptokinase, which worked well enough but caused all sorts of antibody problems. This was followed by a similar enzyme called urokinase, which was not antigenic (antibody stimulating), but which could interfere dangerously with the blood clotting mechanisms. What was wanted was a drug that became activated only when it came in contact with the unwanted clot. Such a drug has now been produced.

Acylated streptokinase-plasminogen compounds (APSAC) have target-seeking properties on the clot in the coronary artery. Angiography (X-ray of a radio-opaque fluid in the blood vessel) has shown that this stuff, given by normal intravenous injection within an hour or two of onset of the coronary, can dissolve the clot and allow the vital re-perfusion of the heart muscle. Note that the drug does not modify the condition of the artery which has led to the clot – it only reverses the last stage in the process, the clotting.

Happily we now have new ways of dealing with coronary narrowing from atherosclerosis, including a method using a tiny balloon to stretch and widen the artery. This is called 'balloon angioplasty' and is another large growth area.

Recombinant DNA techniques ('genetic engineering') are now being used to produce large quantities of materials similar to APSAC. It certainly seems inevitable that this kind of treatment, or a development of it, is going to save a lot of lives in the future.

It is reassuring to know of these new techniques in the treatment of clotting. You will, however, certainly agree that an adjustment in your lifestyle, to avoid the main causes of clots forming, makes much more sense.

5　Smoking

There has been a notable decline in smoking among professional people although many of them still continue to do so. If you are one of these, your attitude to the subject is likely to be ambivalent, perhaps a mixture of concern and of smouldering aggression against those who go on and on about it and probably have no idea what it is like to try to stop smoking. You are likely to think you already know all the facts and have worked up a pretty effective rationalisation about the whole thing.

This chapter assumes that you do not begin to understand the facts, because if you did, the last thing in the world you would ever consider doing would be to put another cigarette in your mouth.

The effects of smoking on the lungs

The cells lining the air tubes in the lungs of a healthy person have a remarkable appearance under a microscope. They are tall 'columnar' cells and the surface nearest the inside of the tube is covered with a multitude of fine hairs which move together, like wind blowing across a field of ripe corn. But the hairs, called 'cilia' are not being blown by the air rushing along the bronchial tube. The movement is spontaneous and carries dust and other foreign material upwards and away from the deeper parts of the lungs. This is one of the body's protective processes. Without it, unwanted material in the inspired air would find its way into the smallest and most

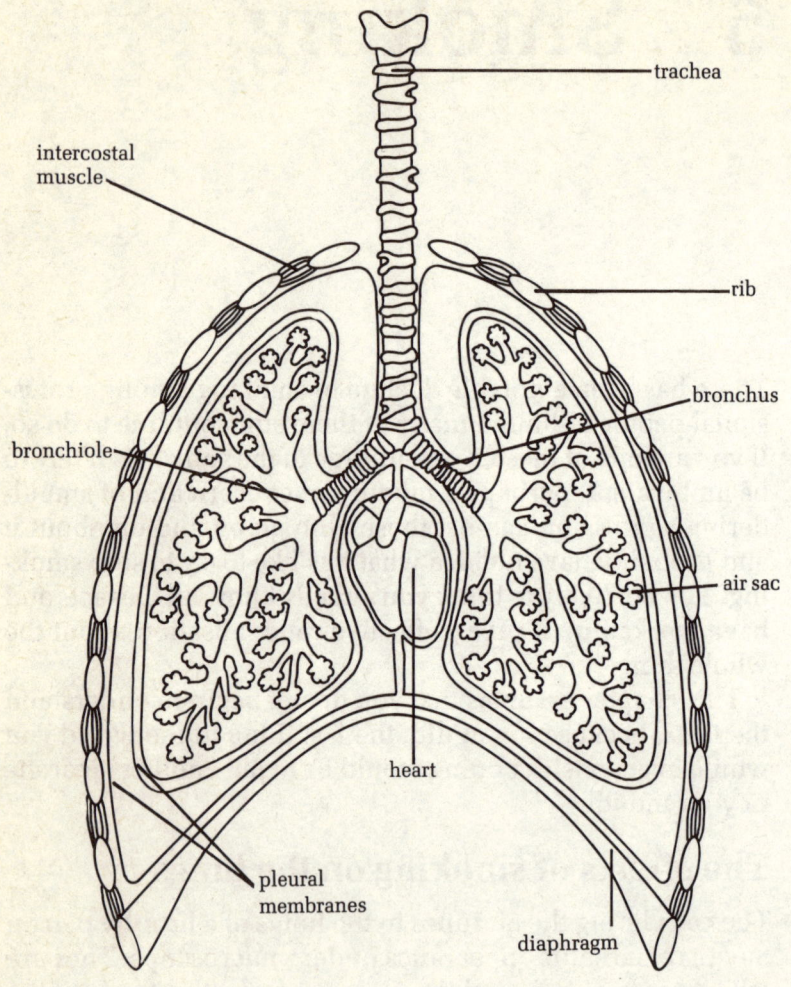

Figure 5 — The Lungs

sensitive air tubes and then into the delicate air sacs where oxygen from the inhaled air is transferred to the blood.

People who smoke cigarettes, soon suffer three obvious changes in these important cells. First, the cilia disappear, then the number of cells increases and finally, the cells become flattened, so that the columnar lining is replaced by a quite abnormal atrophied, scaly layer. After a time there is a tendency for these bald, flattened cells to begin to show signs of excessive multiplication. Some years later this may develop into cancer.

How does lung cancer show itself?

A person with a 'smoker's cough' might notice a change in the sound of the cough, or in its frequency. They may even notice that breathing has become noisy. There may be chest pain and shortness of breath and the sputum brought up when coughing may occasionally be tinged with blood. Soon after this, there may be fever, loss of weight, hoarseness and inability to swallow.

Sometimes the cancer eats into a large lung artery so that death occurs from massive bleeding. More often the symptoms just get progressively worse, with distressing breathlessness from blockage of a main bronchial tube. This is accompanied by sharp chest pain spreading up into the neck and shoulders as the cancer spreads into the upper ribs, spinal column and neck structures. By this time, the situation is hopeless and the sufferer has only a few short weeks or months until death occurs from remote spread of the cancer to the bones, liver and brain.

How common is lung cancer?

Lung cancer is now the commonest cause of cancer death in men, and is the second cause of cancer death in women, after cancer of the breast. In England in 1983, 33,622 people died from cancer of the lung. The ratio of deaths in males compared to females is three to one, but the condition is becoming more common in women because of the considerable increase in smoking by them in the last 30 years. Study after study has shown that the risk of lung cancer is about 20 times greater in smokers than in non-smokers. To paraphrase an excerpt from a leading article in the *British Medical Journal* '. . . tobacco accounts for 15 to 20 per cent of all deaths in Britain. Of every 1,000 young men who smoke, one will be murdered, six will die on the roads, but 250 will be killed before their time by tobacco'.

The more cigarettes smoked, the more marked the early cell changes become. People who have given up smoking have fewer affected cells than smokers, and the number of affected cells becomes progressively less as the number of non-smoking years increases. However, the number of damaged cells never reaches the low level found in people who have never smoked cigarettes. Ironically, there is good evidence that smokers who inhale deeply into their lungs so that the smoke moves quickly past the ciliated cells in the main lung tubes, are slightly less liable to get cancer than those who inhale less deeply. Conversely, the deep inhalers, who carry the smoke right to the air sacs, where some of the constituents enter the bloodstream, suffer a high incidence of coronary thrombosis.

Obviously, every heavy smoker does not get lung cancer. Why is this? For a start, different people show a different tendency to react to the cancer-producing factors in cigarette smoke. Some have very powerful defence mechanisms which can minimise the effects of the tiny smoke particles on the lung tissues. Others have a strong natural, inborn resistance to the typical changes in the cells. 'T' lymphocytes, vital elements in the immune system, exert a kind of cancer surveillance in the body, inspecting abnormal cells for signs of cancer and destroying those which do not meet with their approval. So the state of the immune mechanism is a major factor. A relative deficiency may allow cancer to get a hold if other conditions are promoting it and there is, at present, no practical way of knowing the state of immunological competence in any particular individual.

Lung cancer is not the only form of cancer caused by smoking. Cigarettes are now regarded as the principal known cause of cancer of the larynx, mouth, throat, gullet, pancreas, kidney and bladder. Experts estimate that smoking makes a major contribution in about 30 per cent of all cancers in men and 5 to 10 per cent of cancers in women. The figure for women, is rising.

Smoking and the heart

The evidence linking smoking with heart disease is less direct. We still do not fully understand the mechanism by which smoking causes heart disease. Most of the evidence comes from a series of long-term statistical studies of large population groups, the fate of those whose members' is checked at regular intervals. Some of these groups number over 5,000 people and the studies take into account age, sex, smoking history, blood pressure, weight, amount of physical activity, blood cholesterol levels, stress, family history, the hardness of the local water, and so on.

By finding out what eventually happens to these people and correlating this with the factors mentioned, it is possible to discover which factors are regularly associated with diseases. All the studies show the same result. Cigarette smoking has invariably been found to be a major risk factor in causing coronary thrombosis, stroke and disease of blood vessels generally.

Incidence of the following are all closely related to the number of cigarettes smoked by the subject:

(1) sudden death from heart attack,
(2) coronary artery blockage,
(3) angina pectoris,
(4) stroke,
(5) severe limitation of activity from disease of the blood vessels supplying the legs.

The heavier the smoking the higher the risk. Pipe and cigar smoking apparently do not increase the risk of these conditions. The studies also show that, in those who stop smoking, the increased risk to the heart and blood vessels is reduced by 90 per cent in a period of only 18 months.

What is the link?

Post-mortem examination of the blood vessels of smokers show the characteristic changes of atherosclerosis in the inner layer. Atherosclerosis has already been touched on, but the subject is so important that it warrants more detailed examination.

When the blood vessels of dead smokers are examined, the inner linings instead of being perfectly smooth and even, show irregularity and lumpiness. This is caused by a deposit of fatty tissue and cholesterol just under the surface, mixed up with degenerate muscle cells and elastic connective tissue. The term 'atherosclerosis' comes from two Greek words meaning 'porridge' and 'hardness' and the atherosclerotic plaques usually affect the larger and the medium-sized arteries. Over the years, these plaques tend to grow, and the inner surface of the vessel at that site becomes so altered that blood platelets (tiny bodies important in clotting) coming in contact with it tend to adhere and start the process of coagulation. A very serious state of affairs.

This abnormal clotting of blood within the vessel is called 'thrombosis' and may result in a stoppage of the supply of blood to the tissue which the vessel is feeding. You can appreciate the danger if atherosclerosis affects the coronary arteries of the heart. Unfortunately, this is exactly what does happen, especially to heavy smokers. When one of these arteries becomes blocked the result is sudden death or, if a small branch is involved, a dangerous and disabling illness.

Now it is not being suggested that smoking is the primary cause of atherosclerosis (see Chapter 4). However, there is undeniable evidence that smokers show more atherosclerosis than non-smokers. Also smokers are 20 times more likely to suffer major episodes related to atherosclerosis (coronary thrombosis, angina, stroke, gangrene of the legs) than non-smokers.

Carbon monoxide

Cigarette smoke contains a gas called carbon monoxide which is avidly taken up by the red cells of the blood. The function of these red cells, as already explained, is to take up oxygen in the lungs and carry it to all parts of the body where it is needed to oxidise fuel and release energy. The link between oxygen and the haemoglobin in the red cells is a loose one. The opposite is true when red cells take up carbon monoxide. Here, the chemical bond with the haemoglobin is so strong that carbon monoxide remains in the cell for weeks in the form of the stable compound 'carboxy-haemoglobin'. In this way, part of the haemoglobin of the blood is unavailable for its proper purpose of oxygen transfer. Incidentally, the cause of death in coal gas or car exhaust poisoning is this same carbon monoxide, which has caused a massive conversion of haemoglobin to carboxy-haemoglobin. A 50 per cent dose is fatal.

Heavy smokers can readily achieve carboxy-haemoglobin levels of 5 per cent or even 8 per cent in their red cells. To compensate for the reduced availability of oxygen to the tissues, a 20 per cent increase in blood flow is necessary. Vessels narrowed by atherosclerosis may not be able to do this – with predictable results. To quote one major text-book of medicine, 'Sudden death is the most frequent clinical event associated with cigarette smoking. Cessation of smoking, promptly and sharply reduces the risk of this event'.

What about nicotine?

The significance of nicotine is not clear. Many authorities on the subject consider that none of the risks of cigarette smoking are connected with nicotine. Others are more wary and point out that the nicotine-induced increase in heart rate and raised blood pressure, and the possible constriction of the coronary arteries, are probably contributory. Certainly there is no medical argument over the proposition that patients with coronary artery disease, who continue to smoke, are dicing with death.

Smoking and chronic bronchitis

Chronic bronchitis ('chronic' comes from the Greek word for time and simply means 'going on for a long time') is the condition in which the person concerned coughs up sputum most days, for at least three months of each year – usually the winter months. Most heavy smokers have chronic bronchitis, although they do not call it that. Few of them consult a doctor. 'It is just a smoker's cough' they say. Chronic bronchitis often starts with the inhalation of irritant material, such as cigarette smoke or other air pollutants. As we have seen, such irritants cause interference with the ciliated cells lining the bronchial tubes and eventually destroy the ciliary action altogether. They also stimulate excess mucus secretion from the glands in the air passages and because the cilia are not working properly, this mucus accumulates in the tubes. Irritants, such as tobacco smoke, also interfere with the white blood cell mechanism which combats infection in the lungs. As a result of this, the stagnant material in the tubes becomes infected.

To clear this irritating material from the tubes, the individual has to cough. Often the efficiency of the coughing is impeded by a tendency for the circular muscles in the wall of the bronchial tube to contract, so causing the tubes to narrow. This is called 'bronchospasm' and it causes wheezing. Asthma is a severe form of bronchospasm.

When one considers the habits of the average smoker – sucking into the mouth a great draught of thick smoke, then deliberately drawing the concentrated smoke down into the lungs – it is not in the least surprising that the lungs respond in the way they do. You can hardly imagine anyone doing this with smoke from any other source, such as burning cardboard or wood. Yet smokers deliberately habituate themselves to doing just this and learn to inhibit the resulting coughing.

In the early stages, chronic bronchitis is a comparatively mild disease. With time and continued abuse, it is likely to progress to the very unpleasant condition called emphysema or 'chronic obstructive airway disease'. Here, large numbers of the tiny lung air sacs break down to form a smaller number of larger air spaces. The trouble with this is that the total surface area now available for oxygen transfer to the blood is greatly reduced. As a result the patient becomes short of oxygen, perhaps critically short. In addition, the smaller bronchial tubes become inflamed, narrowed and partially blocked by mucus which cannot get out. The end result may be a constant, exhausting and irremediable state of breathlessness. The unhappy patient, to maintain his laboured breathing, is forced to use his shoulder muscles to try to increase chest movement. His skin may show an ominous blueness and he may, in the final stages of the disease, need to wear an oxygen mask continuously.

Why do people smoke?

There can be very few people unaware, at least in a general way, that cigarette smoking is dangerous and damaging, and yet millions continue to indulge. What makes so many people act so gravely against their own interests?

Many people smoke from the apparently uncontrollable need to give themselves a little 'treat' whenever they feel inclined. It is a pleasant and instantly-available form of gratification and indulgence. Some smokers have said that the cylindrical perfection of the virgin cigarette has a strong aesthetic appeal. For others, there is satisfaction in the mere act of consumption, even in the destruction of something aesthetically pleasing.

The pharmacological (drug) action of nicotine is probably the most important reason for smoking. Many people would probably not bother to smoke were it not for the temporary 'lift' provided. It is a mistake to think that addiction to cigarettes is a genuine pharmacological state, such as occurs in addiction to narcotic drugs. In real addiction, certain cells in the nervous system suffer long term changes so that withdrawal of the drug may be extremely unpleasant. Cigarette smoking causes no such effects and stopping smoking is not associated with any withdrawal symptoms in the pharmacological sense. The claim that smoking is a pharmacological addiction is just another rationalisation adopted to provide an acceptable reason to avoid an undesired course of action.

The impulse to self-gratification is powerful, central and natural. It should be admitted and accepted as one of our major motivating forces. However, the yielding to this impulse should be under the control of the reason. We should be able to distinguish those acts of immediate, short-term gratification which are likely, in the long term, to have gravely ungratifying effects.

The cost of smoking

The National Health Service spends hundreds of millions of pounds every year on treating, or trying to treat, tobacco related diseases. That money is contributed by tax paying smokers and non-smokers alike and would be better applied to purpose of health improvement for all – welfare, medical research, preventive medicine, and so on.

Then there is the cost to society of the loss of productive capacity, working time and trained expertise. Again, all suffer. Finally, we should never forget the cost to individual families in lost income, in the health-sapping effect of having a chronic invalid in the house and in eventual bereavement. That is the true cost of smoking.

How to stop smoking

Motivation is everything, so the first thing to do is to give yourself a sufficiently good reason to stop. A vague, uninformed feeling that you really ought to stop is no good. You must be clearly aware of what you are doing to yourself by continuing to smoke. If you are not by now, then you should go back and read this chapter again. Next, you must put entirely out of your mind any ideas about smoking being a form of drug addiction. It is nothing of the sort.

Cutting down as a means of gradually giving up, is a waste of time and you will never stop that way. Very few people claim to have been helped by substitutes (dummy cigarettes and the like) and it is doubtful if these are of much value. Courses in quitting, group therapy, hypnosis and such activities are for those who merely want to postpone the final decision to stop. Of course it is unpleasant to lose something you have enjoyed for years. Of course, you are going to be irritable and feel deprived, but you must face the issue and make a rational decision about it.

There is only one way to stop. That is to do it right now, in the middle of a packet. Totally, permanently and with the minimum of fuss. Get rid of all cigarettes, air the house, keep away from smokers and learn to enjoy clean living once again.

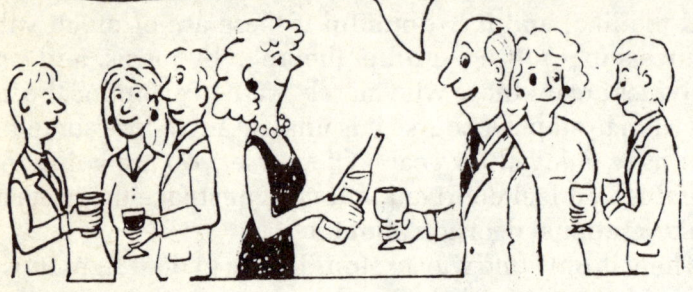

6 Alcohol

The Greek law-giver, Solon, had an excellent maxim for all those seeking health and contentment – *meden agan*. It means 'moderation in everything' and is especially appropriate in relation to alcohol.

Alcohol is a blessing which is very easily abused. The purpose here is to clarify some misunderstandings about it and enlighten you on some important facts so that you can avoid the most obvious dangers to your health.

The warning signs

Am I drinking too much? Are these lunches and drinks after work becoming too excessive? Am I having a drink rather than eating a meal? Do I need a drink in order to cope with stress at work? These are very important questions and, fortunately, we can easily get reliable answers to them. The signs of excessive drinking are clear. If any of the following points apply to you, you are either heading for trouble or already deeply in it.

(1) Drinking is beginning to be a good deal in your thoughts.

(2) It has become an important part of your life, rivalling other major activities.

(3) Your drinking patterns are becoming established and you are drinking every day with a regular indulgence at

lunch time. (Ordinary social drinkers do not have a regular pattern of drinking.)

(4) Undesirable social or legal effects do not deter you.

(5) You have a wonderful head for drink and can carry on 'normally' after an intake that would put the next man under the table. (This means that your nervous system has had a great deal of damaging practice in adapting to high blood alcohol concentrations. It does not indicate a tough, manly ability to 'hold your drink'.)

(6) About ten hours after the last drink you need another one very badly. The mornings are pretty terrible, your hands are shaking, maybe your whole body shakes and you feel sick. Ordinary sounds seem intolerably loud, there is a singing in your ears (tinnitus) and your skin is itching.

(7) There is a marvellous cure for all this – a good stiff drink.

(8) You are no longer able to control your drinking. You just go on until you run out of money, or the barman refuses to serve you.

(9) If you manage to stop for a while, one relapse brings back the whole pattern.

To get yourself into a situation like this takes quite a deal of effort on your part and is not achieved quickly. On average it takes 10 to 15 years to reach a stage of major addiction, but the range may be as wide as 2 to 25 years. So, if you have been drinking moderately all your adult life, are over 35 and in the clear, you can probably congratulate yourself. But do not let that prevent you from noting the warning signs!

How much is safe?

Alcohol consumption is rising steadily in Britain and careful surveys have also shown a progressive rise in the serious liver disease, with all the social and economic damage consequent on alcohol-related loss of ability.

Interestingly, in France where alcoholism is very common and the annual death rate from cirrhosis of the liver is very

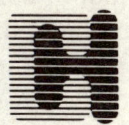

high, there was a striking drop in deaths from this disease during both World Wars when wine was severely rationed.

Alcoholic drinks contain various flavouring substances called 'congeners' and it is these which make brandy taste different from gin. The congeners also have a good deal to do with the severity of the hangover, but it is the ethyl alcohol (ethanol) in all of them that does the real harm. A French study has shown that a daily intake of 80 grams of ethanol, or less, is not very likely to harm the liver. People taking this amount may not be immune from cirrhosis. One person in twenty, in the large group of people with cirrhosis this trial studied, was taking only about 80 grams a day – if they can be believed. Unfortunately, most people find it difficult to admit truthfully just how much they drink. 61 per cent of the people with cirrhosis were drinking more than 160 grams of ethanol per day.

So that you can appreciate what this means, we use the 'unit' system of assessing drink intake. One unit of drink is a half pint of average strength beer (about 3 per cent), a single of 70 degree proof spirit, or one glass of wine. Note that one unit contains eight grams of ethanol. This means that someone drinking 80 grams of ethanol a day is taking about five pints of beer, five double whiskies or a bottle of wine. Table 1 gives some useful information about blood alcohol concentrations in both men and women. Table 2 explains the effects in more graphic details and provides a salutary reminder of the legal position.

Alcohol and the liver

This section should be read with special attention by the female executive, for it is clearly established that women are far more sensitive to the adverse effects of excess alcohol than men.

All alcohol drunk is quickly absorbed and passes in the bloodstream to the liver where the earliest observable effect is a condition known as 'fatty liver'. This causes enlargement of the liver by the deposition of excess fat within the liver

Table 1: Blood alcohol concentrations in mgm per cent.

Average-sized man

Units	At 1 hour	At 2 hours	At 3 hours
1	20	0	0
2	40	10	0
3	60	30	20
4	80	60	40
5	100	80	60
6	120	100	90
7	140	120	110
8	160	150	130
9	180	170	150
10	210	190	170

Average-sized woman

Units	At 1 hour	At 2 hours	At 3 hours
1	30	10	0
2	60	20	10
3	80	40	30
4	110	80	60
5	140	110	80
6	170	140	120
7	200	170	140
8	220	200	170
9	250	220	200
10	300	250	220

Note: the blood concentrations will vary with the weight. The lighter the person, the higher the concentration for a given input.

cells. It is more of a warning than a danger. The various liver functions which are essential to life, usually continue fairly normally. The purely clinical signs of fatty liver are externally indistinguishable from those of alcoholic hepatitis. This is such a serious condition the experts state that, if a patient with a heavy drinking history has an enlarged liver, it is justifiable to perform a liver biopsy in order to be sure.

Table 2: Effects of various blood alcohol concentrations.

Person of average tolerance (moderate drinker)

Blood Alcohol mg %	Effects
20	Feeling good. Little or no effect on performance.
40	Able to 'let go' socially. Slightly dangerous when driving fast.
60	Feeling great! Judgement impaired. Not a time to make important decisions. Driving becoming reckless.
80	Definite loss of co-ordination. Unsafe at any speed. *Legal limit in Britain.*
100	Feeling sleepy. Knocking over drinks.
160	Obviously drunk. Perhaps aggressive and unmanageable. May not remember what happened next day.
300	In coma.
500	Dead.

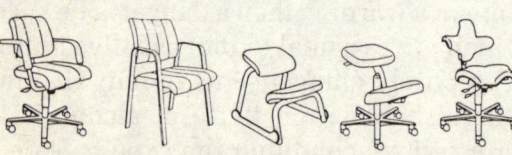

Alcoholic hepatitis can be diagnosed by microscopic examination of the biopsy specimen. This will show areas of cell death and patches of characteristic inflammation. The liver performs so many functions essential to life that severe liver disease is always very serious. People with alcoholic hepatitis often die within two weeks of admission to hospital. They die with deep jaundice (yellow staining of the skin and eyes from retained bile), from liver coma, bleeding into the bowel, kidney failure or severe, uncontrollable infection. As may be imagined, treatment is not particularly effective and the only really useful measure is complete abstinence from alcohol. The only hope then is that sufficient liver cells have survived the onslaught of the ethanol to keep the patient alive.

People who drink enough to cause this condition often eat very little, because they get enough calories from the alcohol to keep them going. Of course, that means they are short of essential amino acids and vitamins (see Chapter 8) and these have to be provided as part of the treatment. There is, however, no medicine that can restore poisoned cells to life.

Cirrhosis is a chronic (in this case, permanent) disease which, if the patient survives, may follow alcoholic hepatitis. It may also occur quietly on its own. This is a condition in which the functional liver cells are killed and replaced by fibrous tissue. The tissue is the same material that closes wounds and binds the edges together, so it is sometimes called 'scar tissue'. The effect of fibrosis on the liver is as if the whole organ were infiltrated by a massive system of fine, criss-crossing scars. These contract to cause distortion and a nobbly appearance. The liver may become much smaller than normal and the number of surviving and functioning liver units will depend on the amount of alcoholic damage. Again, apart from stopping the damage by cutting out alcohol and hoping for the best, there is simply nothing to be done.

Chronic pancreatitis

This condition is basically different from hepatitis in several ways. It is present most commonly in men aged 30 to 45, who are drinking 15 to 20 units a day and taking a rich diet, high in fats and protein. There are episodes of pain, high in the abdomen, spreading through to the back and usually lasting for at least a day. A short period of jaundice usually occurs and an X-ray or CT scan will show that the pancreas is full of cysts, many of them filled with chalky stones. These attacks tend to recur and the pain may be very severe.

Because the pancreas is the only source of insulin in the body, severe damage of this sort is liable to cause diabetes. Other problems may occur, such as damage to the nearby bowel, which may become narrowed or completely blocked. The mortality, in those people who go on drinking after developing chronic calcifying pancreatitis, is very high.

Alcohol and the heart

Alcohol does not directly affect the heart unless a great deal is drunk over a period of at least ten years. So most of the people who get this problem are chronic alcoholics. There are fairly clear indications that the condition is caused, not only by direct alcohol damage to the heart muscle, but also by nutritional and vitamin deficiency in people who get enough calories from the alcohol not to require to eat.

The first sign of trouble is gradually increasing breathlessness on exertion together with palpitation (obvious awareness of the beating of the heart). There is none of the acute chest pain of coronary thrombosis or angina. If medical advice is not sought, the condition progresses to swelling of the ankles and fluid in the chest from failure of the heart to keep a sufficiently good circulation going. The heartbeat becomes irregular, the pulse abnormally fast, and death may occur from severe heart failure.

The ironical thing about alcoholic cardiomyopathy (heart muscle disease) is that if the affected person can be persuaded to give up alcohol completely, even in an advanced stage of the disease, recovery is 100 per cent. Unfortunately, persuasion often fails and victims go back to drinking as soon as they are out of hospital. As with alcoholic liver disease, this is another way to literally drink yourself to death.

Mental effects of alcohol

Excessive drinking is one of the most common causes of mental illness, brought about in two ways. Firstly, by the direct toxic effect of sustained contact between alcohol in the blood and the tissues of the brain and nervous system. Secondly, by the indirect effect on the mind of all the shattering social, sexual and economic effects of alcohol dependency. Here we are concerned with the first group. Typical of this effect is 'alcoholic dementia' which comes on very gradually in heavy drinkers, usually quite late in life. The patient, often female and usually around 60, shows a definite change in personality and severe loss of memory. They may seem either unconcerned or depressed but, on testing, will be found to have suffered severe deterioration in mental powers, with poor judgement and inability to relate socially in the normal way. Likely to deny excessive drinking they may show some cunning in keeping up their intake inconspicuously. A CT scan will show obvious atrophy of the outer layer (the cortex) of the brain. This is the part concerned with the higher functions of the nervous system, including intelligence.

Other effects of alcohol on the brain include the condition of Wernicke's 'encephalopathy' which is due to a severe deficiency of the vitamin thiamine (vitamin B1). Its symptoms include paralysis of the movement of the eyes, severe loss of balance and gross mental confusion. The symptoms occur only after very heavy, prolonged drinking, and treatment, by thiamine injections, is always urgently needed. If a person with Wernicke's encephalopathy does not get medical attention, the condition eventually progresses to a state known as Korsakoff's syndrome. In this state there is the most profound loss of memory, both for recent and remote events, so that the patient can hardly remember anything at all. This may result in the patient inventing fictitious accounts to make up for the defect in memory but quickly forgetting what they have just said. Once Korsakoff's syndrome is established, treatment is almost impossible. Only 14 per cent of sufferers show any improvement, even on the best management, over a period of five years.

Memory blackouts are common in heavy drinkers if the blood alcohol level gets high enough. Moderate drinkers sometimes get them if they over-indulge, but it is usually only the really hardened drinkers who can reach a high enough blood level to cause them. You may be relieved to learn that such lapses are not a sign of alcoholic dementia. Nevertheless, they are a clear warning that you are hitting the bottle far too hard.

Delirium tremens (the 'DTs') is a withdrawal condition occurring up to 72 hours after the last drink. There is clouding of consciousness, then horrifying hallucinations associated with extreme terror, occasional attempts to commit suicide, violently threatening behaviour and disordered action of the heart. The attack, unless effectively treated by injections of powerful sedatives, may go on for as long as five days and the mortality – usually from heart failure – is appreciable.

Chronic alcoholism

The term 'alcoholism' is becoming a little unfashionable and has recently tended to be replaced by the phrase 'alcohol dependence syndrome'. You may be interested to know the official World Health Organisation definition of this syndrome:

A state, psychic and usually physical, resulting from taking alcohol, characterised by behavioural and other responses that always includes a compulsion to take alcohol on a continuous or periodic basis in order to experience its psychic effects, and sometimes to avoid the discomfort of its absence; tolerance may or may not be present.

Note that no reference is made to the physical or mental damage usually associated with alcohol dependence. Also note that there are plenty of people who drink to excess and who do themselves considerable physical and mental damage but who are not, strictly speaking, dependent on alcohol. For that reason, the definition has been criticised and it has been suggested that it ought to include reference to the harmful medical effects.

Here, we are concerned solely with the question of dependence. It is sometimes thought that, as with drugs like heroin, dependence on alcohol will inevitably occur if enough is taken. This, however, does not seem to be so. It is only a comparatively small proportion of drinkers who become chronic alcoholics. In these, the dependence seems very definitely to be psychological rather than pharmacological. Because the treatment of established alcohol dependence is so very difficult it is extremely important to spot the problem early and try to avoid it, but how?

Alcohol dependence is probably always related to a personality problem. It is likely that in most cases the personality problem causes the excessive drinking because of short term gains from alcohol. Alcohol is a great consoler and it may be that you are turning to it to enjoy the state of mind you feel is being denied in your normal life. Perhaps, if you are sufficiently honest with yourself, you may be able to admit that there are elements in your life, which you feel unable to cope with. Elements from which your only apparent relief lies in the effects of alcohol.

A sense of professional or business failure, constant frustration, inability to relate easily to others – all these, and many more, may be indicators of your liability to become permanently dependent on alcohol. If you are aware of any such factors and are worried about your drinking, you should clearly see that you may be gravely at risk of passing into a far worse state – that of chronic alcohol dependence.

How to cope with the threat

Most experts agree that, in contrast with the much simpler case of smoking, it is a complete waste of time to tell someone with a drink problem to stop. It is equally futile to try to frighten them into stopping by recounting horror stories. To do that, without offering anything but blunt insistence on total abstinence, is cruel and pointless and will only deepen depression.

Problem drinkers should, of course, be as fully aware as possible of the medical consequences of their activities. They are not likely to be in any doubt about the social consequences, but vague ideas about the risk to liver and brain are not really enough. Moreover, they should never consider that the matter is out of their hands. Every drinker has some measure of control, but not every drinker wishes to exercise it. One of the aims of treatment must be to provide strong motivation in order to exercise this control.

Problem drinkers need all the help they can get. The first step in obtaining such help is to acknowledge that the problem exists, to accept it and seek immediate help. Alcohol treatment units exist in all major towns and these are run by people who have seen it all, on numerous occasions, and whom nothing will surprise. In most of these units the emphasis is on group therapy, along the supportive lines of 'Alcoholics Anonymous' but with the full gamut of skilled medical and psychiatric resource also available. Problem drinkers attending such units receive specific treatment, not only for the alcohol dependence, but also for any associated nutritional or other secondary effects.

The use of drugs, as a primary measure in the management of alcoholism, is not generally adopted but can be valuable in some cases. The commonest drug used, Disulfiram, has the trade name 'Antabuse'. It is not a very pleasant form of therapy. The drug prevents the acetaldehyde formed from alcohol, from being broken down further into harmless substances, so the acetaldehyde accumulates and makes the patient feel very ill indeed. The effect occurs only if alcohol is taken and is so unpleasant that no one is likely to want to repeat the experience. About five minutes after taking alcohol, the skin flushes and the blood-pressure falls. There is profuse sweating, breathlessness, severe headache, alarm-

SUBSCRIBE TO
GOOD HEALTH
AND GET A *FREE*
STRESS MONITOR CARD

With your first issue of *Good Health* you will also receive a free stress monitor card. The stress monitor card is a fun way of finding out if you, your family or friends are stressed or calm. For those that show stress, there is a simple exercise on the back of the card to help you relax.

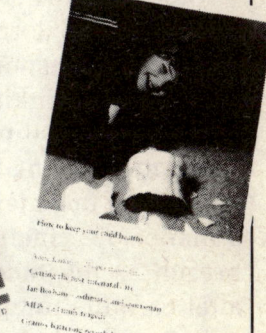

Good Health is about better health for you. Being healthy allows you to lead a rich and full life. This is where *Good Health* can help:

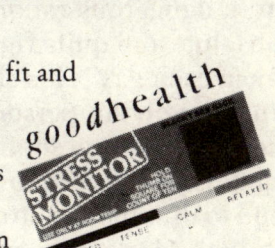

★ Learn how to stay fit and healthy by taking sensible preventative measures and precautions and knowing when to get help if necessary

★ Keep up to date with the latest medical research

★ Learn how to make the best use of medical facilities

★ Feel confident that the information in *Good Health* is reliable and well tested because the Editor is a doctor and the contributors are all experts

★ *Good Health* is good fun too! You will be amused and entertained by the humorous and general interest articles. All this for only £12 per subscription. Your *Good Health* is worth more than this small investment.

ing pain in the chest, nausea and vomiting and sometimes collapse. Antabuse treatment is only ever used in reasonably young, fit people who are made completely aware of the effects. You really have to be determined to want to stop drinking in order to take that 200 mg pill every morning!

Can I help myself?

For the much commoner case of the immoderate drinker who has not degenerated too far, the realistic answer seems to be to make a determined effort to return to moderate drinking. In some ways this is a revolutionary idea and not every doctor agrees with it. Few doctors will, however, deny the futility of just telling heavy drinkers to stop.

Firstly, the drinker must accept that the whole responsibility is his. No external factors (unreasonable demands by the boss, nagging spouse, etc.) may be used as excuses for an increase in drinking. This excuse-making must be recognised for what it is, a dangerous rationalisation. Secondly, there must be an absolute and quite rigid upper limit on the number of units taken each day. This should be regarded as a matter of principle, involving personal honour, and any breach as disgraceful. The limit should be decided upon after careful thought, having regard to the fact that too high a limit will only tend to diminish control. It should certainly not exceed six units in the day and no more than two of these should be taken before the evening. Carrying the allowance over into subsequent days is prohibited. Drinking must be *slow*. Small sips rather than gulps and it is much better to take the units in light beer or wine, rather than in spirits. Remember that some ciders are much stronger than beers and avoid them. If possible, take the units along with a meal in order to delay absorption.

In this battle, winning is so important that you must be ready to receive some 'wounds'. You must be ready to make some radical changes in your lifestyle and habits. It may be necessary to avoid certain drinking companions and pubs. Try to find a good use for the time formerly wasted in drinking. There are plenty of activities which will prove more rewarding. Emotional problems must be looked at squarely and as objectively as possible and discussion with a doctor or psychiatrist can be very helpful.

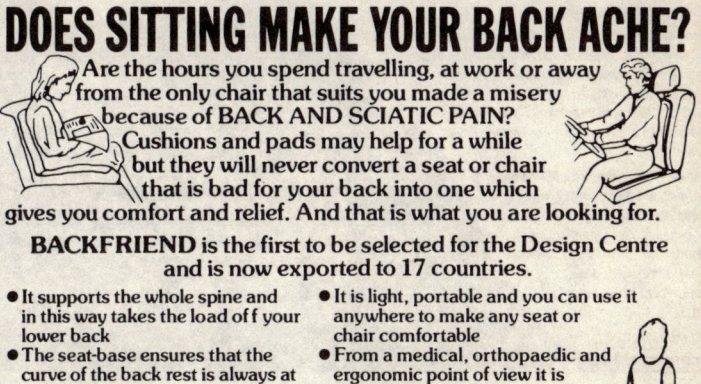

7   Preventive action to stay healthy

'Blessed is the man who lives a mile from the station, for he shall have long life upon the earth. And doubly blessed is he who has a hill between his house and the railway!' Blessed, that is, if he has the sense to take advantage of his good fortune and walk to the station every day. To many, unfortunately, the distance only too readily justifies the use of a car, often on the grounds that time is too valuable to waste on walking. Perhaps you can be persuaded to the contrary.

The body has a great capacity for adaptation to changing physical usage; regular walking over a fixed route, say, to the railway station or up those few flights of stairs, quickly becomes easier. What starts as an exhausting slog causing embarrassing sweating and breathlessness, gradually becomes tolerable and eventually pleasurable. Why is this?

During exercise the heart output, in terms of blood volume pumped per minute, increases. This happens for two reasons. Firstly, an increase in the actual rate of pumping. Secondly, an increase in the strength of the contraction of the heart muscle, so that a greater proportion of the total volume of blood in the chambers of the heart is pumped with each beat. This variable output per beat is called the 'stroke volume'. Therefore, the heart output is the rate multiplied by the stroke volume. At rest, this is something like 70 beats per minute, each beat pumping about 70 ml. An output of about 5 litres per minute. This is roughly the total volume of the blood, so when we are resting the entire quantity goes round each minute.

Note that the heart rate could increase considerably without any increase in output, if the stroke volume were to drop. In other words, if each beat pumped a smaller volume of blood, the heart would have to beat faster to keep up the same output. This faster beating would make greater energy demands on the heart and these demands could only be met fully if the blood supply by the coronary arteries were adequate. If the rate were doubled and the volume halved the heart output would be constant, but the energy required to maintain this output would be considerably increased. This is an important point. It highlights the danger to those with an inadequate blood supply to the heart muscle, when their heart rate is increased by emotional excitement. People in this situation are more liable to suffer angina.

If a heart is deprived of all nerve connections it will continue to beat, but at a much higher rate than normal – usually at about 100 beats per minute. In the normal state two sets of nerves, carrying messages from the brain, control the heart rate. These are the 'sympathetic' nerves, which increase the rate, and the 'parasympathetic' nerves which slow it. Strong stimulation of parasympathetic nerves may even stop the heart altogether for a short time. Normally the parasympathetic impulses predominate, so that the resting heart rate is well below the free-running rate of about 100. The sympathetic nerve endings release adrenaline which acts directly on the heart, speeding it up and increasing the force of the contraction. (Free adrenaline in the circulation, derived from the adrenal glands, also speeds the heart.)

Now these controlling nerves arise from a micro-processor in the stem of the brain. This has data inputs from various places providing it with the information it requires to exert proper control over the heart. The most important source of these input data are stretch sensitive receptors, set into the walls of the major artery of the body (the aorta) and two of its most important branches (the carotids) in the neck. These receptors are complex, branching nerve-endings so arranged that any rise in the blood pressure, which stretches the artery wall, results in nerve impulses being sent to the micro-processor in the brainstem. So a rise in blood pressure, other things being equal, automatically results in a feed-back signal to reduce the heart output.

Many other input stimuli also determine the final controlling signal to the heart and these include oxygen levels in the blood, the individual's state of mind and the perception of an incipient need for activity. It is now an established fact that regular strenuous exercise, operating by way of this feedback system, leads to a definite increase in the stroke volume of the heart and a corresponding drop in the pulse rate. Thus, the cardiac output remains constant with a lowered energy demand on the heart. This is one of the features of fitness and is a state devoutly to be wished for.

The importance of stroke volume is reflected in current trends in the management of patients who have suffered coronary thromboses and survived. In the most up-to-date centres, these patients are out on the sports field, six weeks after their coronary attacks, running long distance races against the clock. Some of them are carrying two-way radios and are having their ECGs monitored. However, the fact that they are doing something which would have been considered not only heretical but also desperately dangerous ten years ago, illustrates how important doctors now consider cardio-respiratory fitness in general, and stroke volume in particular, in the recovery and rehabilitation of coronary patients.

Any physical task, repeated at regular intervals, gets easier. That has been known since the dawn of consciousness. It has also been known, by those who have tried it, that improvement in performance can occur at *any* age. What is new is that we are beginning to understand why. We know that exercise can increase the efficiency of the heart pump and can actually improve the profuseness of the blood supply to the voluntary muscles. Subtler things also happen in the muscles. Muscle cells, like all cells, contain bodies called mitochondria responsible for the chemical processes by which energy is released from fuel. Regular strenuous exercise causes an increase in the number and size of these mitochondria in the muscle cells. Moreover, well exercised muscles use more fat as fuel and less glucose and this can reduce the fat content of the blood and possibly reduce the risk of atherosclerosis.

Exercise has been shown to have value for people with chest disease. We have seen how, by gradual improvement in the efficiency of the heart and the muscles, a given level of physical activity can be achieved with a lowered tendency to breathlessness. This can be a great help to those whose activity is already restricted by respiratory disorder. The same has been shown to apply to patients with angina and restricted blood supply to the leg muscles where walking causes pain. Carefully graded exercise can increase the amount of work done before the pain starts.

Keeping it up

Another important fact, now fully accepted, is that the plasticity in the body's adaptive response to use, works both ways. You may achieve a splendid state of fitness by devoted daily exertion and be glowing with health and vitality on the first of April. Give it up and return to your normal torpor, and by the middle of May you will be back where you started. Six sedentary weeks are enough to return you firmly to square one and cut your exercise tolerance to its former feeble standard. Even the level of inactivity has a bearing on your fitness. It is now well known that lying in bed, beyond the statutory seven or eight hours a night, is a highly dangerous habit. Most patients confined to bed by illness take a good deal longer to return to their former level of fitness than the length of the time actually spent in bed. Even young people take at least as long. In the past many elderly patients treated for strokes or other major conditions have been left in bed so long that they have never recovered their former muscular and cardio-respiratory levels, in spite of a complete recovery from the specific disorder. This kind of disability should now be a thing of the past, but we can learn an important lesson from it.

Keeping fit has to become a *permanent* feature of our lives. It is common knowledge that young athletes who give up exercise tend to put on fat. This is obviously because of the continuance of eating habits which are now in excess of the energy demands of the body. What is not so well known is that the figures show that these people are more liable to heart disease than those of us who have never engaged in athletic activity.

Psychological effects of exercise

Anyone who has ever tried regular exercise will confirm that it makes you feel better. Doctors are beginning to discover that patients with mild to moderate depression, in whom drug treatment has failed, may be cured by exercise alone. Several factors may account for the effect of exercise on the mind and no doubt you can work out some of them for yourself. The importance of recognising the close inter-relationship of mental and bodily function has been stressed. It is hardly surprising, therefore, that an increase in the general efficiency and ease of function of one should be reflected in a more healthy function of the other. Awareness of growing physical powers; increase in the capacity for action; the sense of well-being; pride in performance; improved oxygen supply to the brain; loss of embarrassment over physical deficiences, these are all factors which you would naturally expect to improve general equanimity.

There has been much talk recently, of the effects of 'endorphins' (natural morphine-like substances produced by the body during exercise) in causing people to get 'hooked' on strenuous exercise. Endorphins and the similar enkephalins certainly induce a state of euphoria and it seems likely that, for some people, regular long-distance running is addictive.

The management of stress

The elements of this topic are covered in Chapter 3. Refresh your memory and then try to determine your personality type. If you are a 'B' type person, read no further. If you are an 'A', try to analyse in detail the factors causing stress and, in particular, look deeply into your character for signs of repressed hostility. Analyse its nature and determine what prompts it in you. This is the major danger. Do not indulge it. It is a luxury you cannot afford, however eminently justified you may think you are in doing so. Hostility is deadly for you and must be conquered.

Study your own body language. Do your postures reflect stress? Remember that the mind and the body react so closely on each other that a deliberate change in body posture can influence the state of the mind. Interestingly, you will find yourself studying your colleagues, your business contacts, even your interviewees.

This brings us to therapeutic relaxation. This is not just idle lazing. Relaxation is a deliberate technique for undoing the somatic response to stress and conditioning the mind to reject the elements which cause it. Surprisingly, you may find relaxation difficult. If so, you might benefit from classes in relaxation held regularly in most urban centres. It is worth first making the effort to achieve effective relaxation on your own.

This technique should be practised every day, preferably at a time set apart for the purpose. Choose a quiet place where you are unlikely to be disturbed. Before you start, try to dispose of any worrying tasks that might distract you. Lock the door, pull the curtains, dim the lights, if you prefer it. Find a comfortable position, either lying flat or sitting back in a chair. Close your eyes and practice breathing properly – slowly and very deeply so that your abdomen moves out on inspiration. As you breath out, feel the tension 'escaping'. Do not force the breathing. Keep you shoulders down. Relaxation cannot be forced, you must just let it happen. Do not react to thoughts about anything outside your body. Observe the state of various muscle groups in turn and let the tension go. Some people find it helpful to start with the toes and work systematically upwards.

You may need a lot of practice before you master this valuable technique.

Other factors

Apart from exercise and the avoidance of stress, healthy living requires some prohibitions and a lot of respect for moderation. The chief prohibitions are contained in Chapters 5 and 6. The great principle of moderation in everything, is commended to you but whether you will be able to conform to it is another matter. A perusal of Chapters 5, 6 and 8 may help to provide you with the necessary motivation.

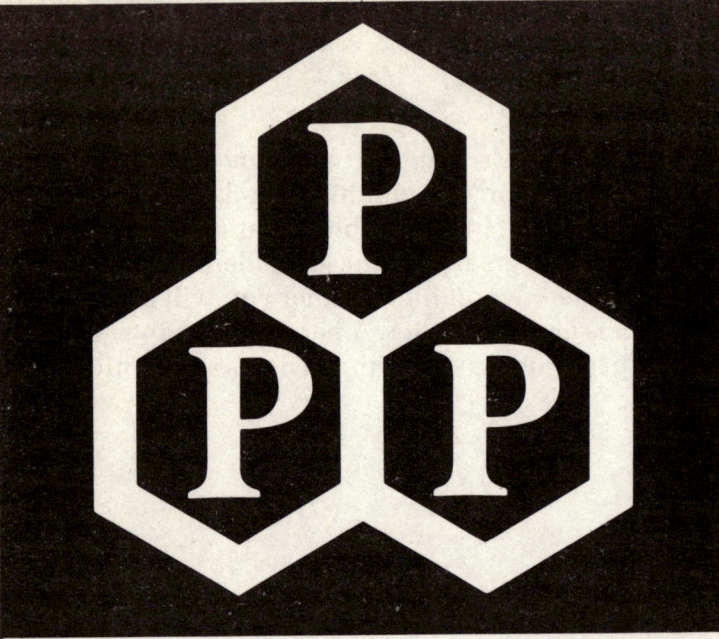

8 A healthy eating plan

Nutrition and health must inevitably be a matter of concern to the busy executive, whose pattern of life constantly puts him in the way of over-indulgence. Like millions in our Western society, he suffers from malnutrition. This is not in the conventional sense of inadequate food intake, but in the sense that the kind and quantity of food eaten is seriously damaging. Many executives are, quite rightly, deeply worried about this.

You should be aware that your excessive intake is simply the result of your uncontrollable inclination to self-gratification. You have also probably recognised that this is such a fundamental need that you would do almost anything rather than abandon the tendency.

So you need advice – strongly persuasive advice – and you have probably already looked for it in other books, where you will not have found any lack of choice. This is a subject of unfailing interest and many of the books produced on diet and health are soundly based and helpful. Unfortunately this subject also attracts many which are not and it is important to be able to distinguish between the two.

Even recommended diets should be looked at with some suspicion, for many of them, some apparently respectable, are based on defective premises. One of the commonest of these is the proposition that rapid weight loss is desirable. It has been shown time and time again that rapid weight loss discourages the establishment of new eating habits. Any weight loss, however great, achieved without this funda-mental requirement is a futile exercise.

Nutritional requirements for health

The body needs fuel as a source of energy and this must be provided, as with any other machine, in accordance with the amount of work done. An average sized man (70 Kilogram) needs about 70 Calories per hour if he is lying back in an armchair watching TV. If he is cutting down trees with an axe, he will require up to 600 Calories an hour. If a lumber-jack retires and proceeds to spend his time in an armchair watching TV, but continues to eat the amount that kept his weight constant when he was working, he will soon get very fat. It is an elementary medical fact that, if a dietary calorie intake is constant, then weight will either be gained or lost according to the amount of muscular work done. In practice it is found that if the calorie input is inadequate, people tend automatically to reduce their physical activity to avoid, if possible, loss of weight.

It is very difficult to lose weight by taking extra exercise. The amount of work that must be done to achieve even a small weight loss is considerable, and very little extra food intake will cancel all the hard-won advantage. Extra exercise also improves appetite so there is a strong incentive to allow that little extra food.

What is a Calorie?

Chemical energy locked up in a fuel can, when released, per-forms work. This is what happens when petrol is burned in a car engine. The fuel is combined with oxygen from the air and energy becomes available. The same kind of thing hap-pens in the body and in this case, the appropriate fuel, is glu-cose derived from the food. Food is chemically processed, mainly in the gut, and the resulting glucose is oxidised, releasing energy. Do not confuse this idea with the purely psychological notion of 'energy' in the sense of having the inclination to be up and doing. Here, we are concerned with a strict definition of energy as the capacity of a body to do work. Some of the energy released by the oxidation of food is used mechanically in muscle contraction, some electrically in the generation of nerve impulses, but most appears as heat. Of course, without food fuel, we would eventually become rather permanently cold.

It is convenient to assess the energy potential of food in terms of heating effect and this is where calories come in. A calorie is the amount of heat needed to raise the temperature of 1 gram of water by 1 degree centigrade. In the context of nutrition that is an inconveniently small unit, so it is multiplied by 1,000 and called a kilocalorie or, usually, just Calorie with a capital 'C'. There is a movement to replace the Calorie with the Joule, which is the standard unit of work, energy and heat. Very roughly, a Calorie is equal to about 4 Joules. Three classes of food material provide energy. These are carbohydrates (4 Calories per gram), fat (9 Calories per gram) and protein (4 Calories per gram).

Carbohydrates and fats

Carbohydrates (cereals, sugars, bakery products, starchy foods, potatoes) are normally the main fuel source, but the calorie requirement could easily be provided by proteins or fats. Such a diet would not be very palatable, but it would not do any great harm to get all the needed calories in this way. Fats give more than twice the number of calories, weight for weight, as carbohydrate or protein. It is a very concentrated fuel source and is popular with heavy manual workers. The actual biochemical necessity for fat is very small indeed. All we require is a tiny quantity of one of the three principle fatty acids (linoleic acid, linolenic acid or arachnidonic acid). It is virtually impossible to avoid getting the small quantity required, unless on a starvation diet.

These three fatty acids, incidentally, are polyunsaturated fatty acids and it seems appropriate to explain this widely used but little understood term. When carbon atoms link to each other and to the atoms of other elements to form the complicated molecules of organic compounds, each is capable of linking to four other atoms. If they link up so that all four 'bonds' connect the carbon atom to four other separate atoms, then the compound formed is said to be 'saturated'. If, however, some of the carbon bonds are not individually used, but link up as double bonds, the compound is said to be 'unsaturated'. Double bonds are actually weaker than single bonds, and saturated compounds are generally more stable than unsaturated.

Dietary fats consist of fatty acids connected, in groups of three, to a glycerol base to form a compound called a triglyceride. Fatty acids may have saturated or unsaturated bonds. Saturated fatty acids are stable fats, like suet, often solid at moderate temperatures. Unsaturated fats will not solidify until much lower temperatures are reached. Fish oils, of course have to remain liquid at quite low temperatures so they are unsaturated as are most plant food oils. The 'poly' just means 'many' and this simply indicates that many of the bonds in these triglycerides are unsaturated. A relative increase in the intake of polyunsaturated fatty acids results in a decrease in the level of the dangerous forms of cholesterol in the blood.

Protein

Although proteins (meat, beans, eggs, dairy products) are an important source of calories, they are also a rather special group in that a severe deficiency does cause disease. There is a good deal of protein in the body's structure, especially in the muscles, and proteins are made up from several smaller building molecules called amino acids. The body can synthesise most of these itself, but there are eight which it cannot manufacture and these must be provided, ready made, in the diet. These eight are called the 'essential' amino acids. Understandably enough, the need for calories always takes priority over constructional requirements. If therefore the calorie intake is inadequate, even the essential amino acids will be used for fuel. Severe shortage of protein in the diet is

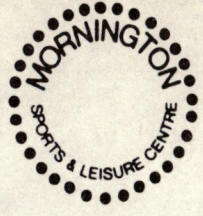
a serious matter and even if there is plenty of fat or carbohydrate, inadequate protein intake will lead to muscle wasting because wear and tear is not being made up.

The daily protein requirement for healthy people is remarkably constant. From the age of about 15 onwards, males require about 55 grams and females about 45 grams.

Vitamins

Vitamins essential for health are the four fat-soluble vitamins, A, D, E and K and the water-soluble vitamins C, Riboflavine, Thiamine, Nicotinic Acid, B6, B12, Biotin, Folacin and Pantothenic Acid. Any reasonably mixed diet will contain far more than the minimum requirements of these vitamins, and some of them are so widely distributed in food that deficiency has not been demonstrated. Table 3 shows adequate daily intake and Table 4 gives the sources.

Table 3: Adequate daily vitamin requirements for adults.

Amounts in milligrams

Vitamin A	1.0		
Vitamin D	0.01 *	Thiamine	1.5
Vitamin E	10.0	Riboflavine	1.7
Vitamin K	0.1	Niacin	20.0
Vitamin C	60.0	Pantothenic a.	5.0
Vitamin B6	2.2	Folacin	0.4
Vitamin B12	0.003	Biotin	0.1

* That is, 400 international units.

Table 4: Sources of Vitamins.

Vitamin A	Milk, butter, eggs, yellow vegetables, fish liver oil (especially cod and halibut).
Vitamin D	Milk, butter, egg yolk, fish liver oils.
Vitamin E	Seed oils, nuts, beans.
Vitamin K	Liver, cabbage, spinach, tomatoes.
Vitamin C	Citrus fruit, tomatoes, green vegetables, potatoes.
Riboflavine	Milk, eggs, fruit, meat, liver.
Thiamine	Eggs, cereals (whole grain), pork, bananas, apples.
Nicotinic Acid	Liver, milk, tomatoes, leafy vegetables, peanut butter.
Vitamin B6	Whole grain cereal, milk, eggs, fish, liver, yeast.
Vitamin B12	Liver, kidney, milk, eggs, cheese.
Biotin	Liver, eggs, milk (The body makes this vitamin, so do not worry about it.)
Folacin	Liver, fresh leafy green vegetables.
Pantothenic Acid	Egg yolk, lean meat, milk.

Vitamins are of quite fundamental importance to health if they are deficient in the diet. Their presence, in very small quantities, is essential for some of the most basic biochemical functions. Equally, their absence causes serious disease, such as:

(a) corneal softening and perforation (deficiency of Vitamin A),

(b) severe skin, mouth and tongue disorders (deficiency of Riboflavine),

(c) intestinal disturbance, mental depression and paralysis (deficiency of Nicotinic Acid),

(d) neuritis and severe fluid retention (deficiency of Thiamine),

(e) anaemia, debility, gum disorder, mouth ulcers (deficiency of Vitamin C),

(f) softening and distortion of bones (deficiency of Vitamin D).

There is not, and never has been, a scrap of evidence that taking any vitamin in excess of the amounts needed to prevent these disorders can, in any way, improve normal corneas, skin, gums, bones etc. Nor is there any evidence that vitamins give extra energy or confer any other advantage whatsoever.

Dangers of excess vitamin intake

Two vitamins, taken in excess, can cause harm. Excess Vitamin A can cause toxic symptoms such as severe headache, drowsiness and vomiting. If dosage is continued, there may be enlargement of the liver and spleen. Excess intake of vitamin D is even more dangerous. This leads to excessive calcium in the blood with deposition of calcium in joints, kidneys, heart muscle, lungs, skin and even in the corneas. In severe cases the bones may become seriously weakened by calcium loss.

Minerals

Certain minerals are essential, but again, normal reasonably mixed diets will always contain enough. You need Calcium and Phosphorous in fair quantity for bones and teeth, to ensure that the blood clots properly and that the nervous system works as it should. Iron is important for the blood, a little Iodine is needed for the thyroid gland, Magnesium is essential for various biochemical processes and traces of Copper are also required. The need for other minerals, such as Zinc,

Manganese, etc. is not so easy to prove, but it is probable that they are required. The amounts needed, however, are so minute that anyone who eats anything at all will certainly get enough. Table 5 shows the requirements.

Table 5: Adequate daily mineral requirements for adults.

Amounts in milligrams

Calcium	800.0		
Phosphorus	800.0	Copper	2.0
Magnesium	350.0	Manganese	3.0
Iron	10.0	Chromium	0.1
Iodine	0.15	Zinc	15.0

Note: women need 50 per cent to 100 per cent more during pregnancy and lactation.

Obesity

Many sets of weight tables relate weight to height and age, but this merely reflects the fact that most people get heavier as they get older. Of course, this should not happen. Table 6 gives some useful guidelines for acceptable weight range for grown men and women, and you will note that age is not included. The range, for each height, should correlate with the type of body build. Only broad, burly people should reach the upper limit, in each case.

Obesity is usually defined as a body weight of more than 20 per cent over the average ideal weight for the sex and height. People whose weight is more than 30 per cent over the ideal, begin to show excess mortality, a raised incidence of heart disease, high blood pressure, diabetes and other serious conditions. There is no individual fixed point at which these effects begin to appear, but statistics clearly show that after the 30 per cent point they increase continuously in proportion to the excess rise in weight.

Some of us are fated from childhood to be obese and this is a recognised clinical pattern. People with 'lifelong obesity' usually have normal birth weight but become heavy when

Table 6: Acceptable weight range.

Height (Ft)	(Ins)	Men Range (lbs)	Women Range (lbs)
5	0	106-135	96-125
5	1	109-138	99-128
5	2	112-141	102-131
5	3	115-144	105-134
5	4	118-148	108-138
5	5	121-152	111-142
5	6	124-156	114-146
5	7	128-161	118-150
5	8	132-166	122-154
5	9	136-170	126-158
5	10	140-174	130-163
5	11	144-179	134-168
6	0	148-184	138-173
6	1	152-189	142-177
6	2	156-194	146-181
6	3	160-199	–
6	4	164-204	–

quite small children and put on a great deal of weight around puberty. These unfortunates tend, often in spite of great efforts, to return to what seems to be their constitutional state and often become grossly obese later in life.

However, most of us experience only 'adult-onset' obesity. This occurs when we allow the eating habits from our more energetic adolescence and early adult days to persist into the more sedentary middle years. Interestingly, this kind of weight gain ('middle-aged spread') is confined mainly to the centre of the body, whereas life long obesity affects the extremities also. Unsatisfactory eating habits are established in childhood, often in infancy. Early childhood overeating leads to life long obesity for many.

It is common for obese people to blame their 'glands' –

meaning the endocrine organs such as the pituitary and thyroid – for their obesity. In fact, only one case in a hundred is caused in this way. It is true that obesity is often associated with a lack of proper hormone balance, but this is nearly always the result of the obesity, not the cause. One of the most important consequences of obesity is the need for more insulin to control glucose usage by fat and muscle cells. In the end, as weight continues to increase, the available insulin supply is unable to meet the demand and the person becomes diabetic. Heart disease, atherosclerosis, high blood pressure, disease of the lungs, fatty liver and gallstones are also among the unhappy catalogue of disorders which it can cause.

Treatment of obesity

Extra weight is stored entirely as fat. A 25 per cent gain in weight means a doubling of the fat stores. After early adult life, very little of the weight gain represents increased muscle or other tissue. The fuel reserves in the body are exclusively of fat and an average man will store 120,000 Calories – about 70 days' supply. On reducing calorie intake below the metabolic requirements, fat stores immediately begin to be depleted. You cannot do this without feeling hungry. So, if you do not feel hungry you are not losing weight. Only when all the fat stores are gone will the body begin to use up muscle as fuel, but this will not happen if the minimum calorie food intake is supplied. Only in prolonged starvation or disease will the muscles waste.

People with adult-onset obesity have little cause for complaint. For them, the matter is easy – reduce calorie intake. If you are serious and really intend to do what you know you ought to, you will resolve to form new and healthier eating habits. You will simply eat less of everything and, for a time, stoically endure the ensuing pangs of hunger.

The one simple and central necessity for weight loss, is to establish for yourself new, smaller eating habits and a normal, balanced diet with *nothing* between meals. It is as simple as that. If you can also manage to increase your average regular amount of exercise, that will do you a power of good but it will *not*, in itself, lead to weight loss.

At present, drugs to suppress appetite or to increase metabolism do not have any major role in the treatment of obesity. Some are dangerous, others have a very temporary or minor effect. Since the control of weight has to be a life long concern and the only real solution is the formation of new eating habits, drugs which purport to eliminate the need for action on the part of the patient are essentially counter-productive.

The mortality rate in severe obesity is substantial. At age 45, men who are 30 per cent overweight have a 40 per cent higher mortality than those of normal weight. Some doctors have felt justified in arranging to have their patients' teeth wired together to prevent ingestion of solids. In other cases, patients have undergone surgical operations to bypass a large loop of the intestine so that the amount of food absorbed is greatly reduced. The results have not been good

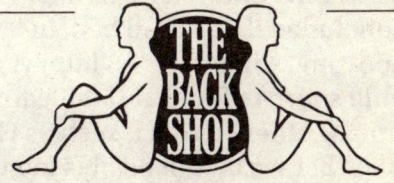
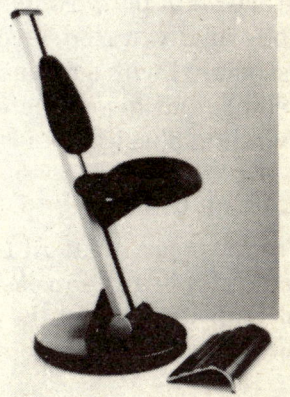
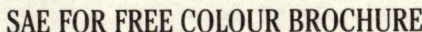

and many complications have occurred, some of them serious. Some plastic surgeons advocate the slicing or sucking of great quantities of fat from under the skin. Even such extreme measures are liable to fail and there is a strong tendency for the remaining fat cells to enlarge to compensate.

Rules for healthy eating

(1) Remember that you are establishing new habits.
(2) For home consumption, buy your own food and avoid those which especially tempt you.
(3) Put small portions on your plate.
(4) Eat slowly. Chew thoroughly, swallow, and pause before taking the next bite.
(5) Enjoy every mouthful.
(6) If at home, throw away leftovers.
(7) Never eat between meals.

Cholesterol

There is much said about cholesterol in Chapters 4 and 5 and you may have concluded that it is all bad. In fact, cholesterol is an essential body ingredient. It is an important constituent of cells, a valuable source of fuel and the parent compound for the production of other steroids, such as Cortisol. So we need cholesterol. What we do not need is too much of it.

The essential fact is that the rate of production of cholesterol by the liver, is closely related to the degree of obesity, so overweight people always have too much cholesterol. Since abnormally raised levels of blood cholesterol are closely associated with serious and irreversible disease of the blood vessels and heart, there would seem to be a good case for avoiding obesity.

Choice of food

We have seen that all the energy and biochemical requirements for health can easily be met by adherence to a few simple rules. Also that the commonest form of malnutrition in the western world is overeating. Our nutritional requirements can be met by an enormous variety of foods but there is a general opinion amongst members of the public that certain foods are, in an unspecified way, 'good for you' and that others are positively harmful.

Unfortunately, the phrase 'good for you' does not really mean very much. To a starving man, any kind of food would be 'good for him'. To a person suffering from a particular vitamin deficiency, an item of food rich in that vitamin would be exceedingly 'good for him'. In the case of people with normal dietary intake, the notion that certain foods have some sort of magical properties to improve health, is questionable. All the food we eat, whatever its origins, passes through the same digestive process with pretty much the same end product.

From time to time anxiety arises about diets being over-rich in one particular ingredient. Refined sugar, for instance, has been described as 'pure white and deadly'. Much has also been made of the over-refinement of many modern 'junk' foods, with inadequate roughage, excess sweetening, and so on. Obviously, concern is appropriate and an informed and critical attitude to what the foodstuff manufacturers are doing, is very much in your interest. You certainly do not want to be eating unasked for antibiotics, anabolic steroids and sex hormones just so that livestock and poultry production is facilitated. Equally, you should not be driven into a kind of anorexia by refusing to eat anything which has not come straight out of virgin soil. The vast food requirements of the modern world simply could not be met without modern farming methods.

Certainly, our bodies were evolved to cope with a simpler kind of nutritional input. Agreed, we eat a hundred times as much sugar as the cavemen did and a great deal less roughage. Unquestionably, it is valuable to bear in mind the kind of primitive environmental and social conditions in response to which our present nutritional physiology evolved. So, if you have a choice between 'natural' and 'junk' food, it is obviously better to select the former. But remember that, because of the way your digestive system works and because of its remarkable capacity for internal adaptation, you body really can, given half a chance and no abuse, do a great job of looking after itself.

9 Keeping fit

The theory of keeping fit was mentioned briefly in Chapter 7. By now you should, hopefully, have a clear picture in your mind of the priorities you must subscribe to in your lifestyle if you are going to avoid shortening, or damaging the quality of it. Your heart may be no more than a rather elegantly controlled and highly efficient mechanical pump, but it is a pump you are critically dependent on, and if it breaks down, nothing else matters at all.

Now we come to the nub of the matter and this could be where the trouble starts. It may be the case that walking to the station every day means adding perhaps half an hour to your already considerable daily travelling time. Time which already eats into the precious and very limited ration available for leisure or – admit it – homework. True you have an extremely tight, busy schedule with very little time to relax and 'recharge your batteries' for the next day's labours. In spite of all that, you now have to consider the suggestion that even walking to the station every day is not enough. That, in addition to all the walking and office stair-climbing, you should also devote ten or twelve minutes every day to the exclusive business of exercising to keep fit.

But, you object, you already give more time than you can afford to fitness, are too old for that sort of nonsense and refuse to make an exhibition of yourself. Furthermore, you would certainly do yourself an injury and might even put your blood pressure up enough to give yourself a stroke.

However, consider the following questions, and their answers.

Is it your wish to achieve something like your natural life-span? And to enjoy it? If so, then the probability is that unless you amend your present way of life, you lessen your chances of doing so.

Is your general state of mind one of boredom, frustration, unhappiness? Do you feel you lack the ability to meet challenge? Is life tedious? Is your temper usually on a short fuse? Do you feel constantly fatigued? If so, then the probability is that your state of fitness is well below par.

Are you self conscious about your appearance – your bulging tummy, the fat pads on your hips, your flabby legs? If so, do you think it better to conceal them or to do something about it?

Do you contantly suffer from backache? If called upon to do anything slightly more strenuous than normal are you liable to do yourself an injury? If so, you are likely to be in a dangerously unfit state. You are at a minimum functional fitness level. Your body has adapted, as bodies inevitably will, to the minimal demands normally made upon it and it has become fit for nothing more.

Now consider the word 'fitness'. Fitness for what? It would be ridiculous to exercise to the point where you were able to snatch 300 lbs or pull a bus with your teeth. These things are possible, but only for those who find them important enough to devote their whole time to them. You need to be fit for life and life ought to include a good measure of all those things the body was evolved to do such as running, walking, lifting, carrying, and so on.

You may object that these things are all right for the young, that evolution operated on the basis that most people would be dead by the age of 30. Well, that is a cogent argument, but it is also an effective basis for rationalising your idleness. For the implication that it is somehow unnatural for older people to try to behave like the young, simply is not true. This is a cultural development. We *allow* ourselves to get old, because it is considered right, proper and dignified to do so.

Conforming to stereotypes of the elderly could be considered to be respectable suicide. Happily, there are plenty of examples of people who have refused to do this.

The standard response

People who read books of this sort, people like you, the executives who want to be healthy, do not need to be told when you are unfit and need to do something about it. You would not be reading this if you were not already concerned. The chances are that you are already familiar with, and thoroughly disillusioned by, the standard response. This response is determined by natural pragmatism and your reaction when you see a problem is to go straight out to solve it, as quickly as possible. You want a crash programme, an instant solution.

Well you may be clear about the existence of the problem, but you also need advice on how to tackle it. Crash programmes are no good in this context. All you get from a crash exercise programme are sore muscles, strained joints and a powerful disincentive to try again. With dieting, the outcome is a month of misery, a week or two of blissful slimness and then a speedy relapse into your former flabby state. The body does not work on crash programmes. Adaptations are achievable – enormous adaptations – for the power to adapt is one of the most striking and biologically advantageous properties of the body. Real adaptation, however, can never occur quickly and the attempt is invariably painful.

So forget the standard crash programme response. This chapter will guide you in making the adaptation at a proper gradual rate. But no adaptation, major or minor, will persist unless the factors causing it also persist. That is really what adaptation means. The whole thing is a constant, dynamic, responsive process. Your fitness level will be a response to what you put into it. If, unhappily, you revert to your former state of idleness, the result is appreciable only over a period of about six weeks. So, make the decision now. If you are serious and are well enough motivated to take on this life-amending programme, read on. But do remember that this is for life.

The hazards of exercise

Of course there are risks, but they are easily avoided so long as you know about them and understand their nature. So this section is important. Above all, please note that if you are over 35 years of age or are in any doubt about the safety of undertaking graded exercise as recommended in this chapter, consult your doctor first. Whilst he cannot give you a cast-iron guarantee that you will never suffer a heart attack when exercising, he will be able to find any objective signs of heart disease and advise you accordingly. His advice will, almost certainly, include the prescription of exercise.

Let us try and get the matter of the danger to your heart into perspective. Just under 10 per cent of fatal heart attacks occur in people while engaged in heavy exertion. In most, it not all, of these cases the exertion will have been unaccustomed. Activities like clearing snow from a path, or pushing a stalled car. Few of those people will have had a fitness level appropriate to the exertion and so they will have required of their hearts a greater work-load than can readily be supplied. Some may even have experienced angina-type pain before the coronary thrombosis came on.

There is no particular reason to suppose that it was the 'heart strain' from the hard work that caused the thrombosis. The following statistics throws some light on this. Some 13 per cent of fatal heart attacks occur while the person concerned is fast asleep in bed. Quietly asleep, under no strain, with the blood flowing gently and sluggishly through the coronaries, ready to clot at any moment. Compare that with the same person engaged in heavy exertion. Then, the blood pressure is up and the coronary flow is at its fastest. About 40 per cent of fatal heart attacks occur when people are just standing and talking. No exertion, no excitement. So you see that there is a fair mythology on the subject, based on lack of data and a misunderstanding of the physiology.

The hazards to the skeletal, muscle and joint systems are much more real. Concern has been expressed by orthopaedic, sports medicine and accident specialists about the rising incidence of problems, some permanent, caused by injudicious exercise. Attention is increasingly being drawn to the high incidence of knee injuries, stress fractures of the foot bones, especially the long bones behind the toes and the heel bone from pavement pounding. Even the shin bone can suffer a stress fracture from heavy and prolonged jogging. Soft tissue injuries are even more common, but being less serious attract less attention. The disability from them can be considerable, however.

All of this extensive experience teaches the same lesson – a lesson the Greeks (who also went in for Marathon races) knew all about. 'Meden agan' is Greek for 'Crash programmes are out. If you do not take it gently and gradually, you are going to suffer'. The literal translation, 'Moderation in everything' does not mean that you should take only a little exercise. It does mean that you must get into exercise little by little. Any exercise scheme which fails to take this into account should be avoided.

The importance of sleep

Sleep needs vary considerably from person to person. It is probable that most of us spend longer in bed than we need, but that is not the same thing as saying that we get enough sleep. It is known that the requirement decreases with age and that disturbed, or intermittent, sleep is the pattern in older people. There is no evidence that this is harmful. If, however, the normal pattern for the individual is disturbed, this will affect the daytime performance and the capacity for work and full living. Although the physiology of sleep is not yet well understood, its necessity is obvious and the effects of deprivation apparent to all. It may be said that the brain needs rest, just as the body does, and that this is provided by sleep.

Sleep disorders are common and some of them have obvious causes. Recurrent nightmares, for instance, result from major unresolved conflicts and are more likely after excessive fatigue, during feverish illnesses and after large alcohol intake. The remedy is to resolve the conflicts and avoid the exacerbating factors.

Insomnia takes various patterns. Initial insomnia, or difficulty in getting off to sleep, is often caused by anxiety or depression. The pattern of early morning waking, with the inability to fall asleep again, frequently occurs in deeply worried, overworked individuals who fall asleep from sheer exhaustion. In this pattern of early morning wakefulness there is often a marked and unjustified magnification of the gravity of current problems, with an abnormal tendency to self-reproach and self-punishment.

Insomnia of both types often results from causes which fully justify the sleep disturbance – worry about work, or marital disharmony, serious concern about health, etc. In such cases, the remedy is not a sleeping pill, but a direct facing up to and resolution of the problem.

Exercise in daily life

To be at a minimum fitness level adequate for your carefully controlled, sedentary lifestyle, really is not good enough. Apart from the long term risks, you have no reserve in hand for emergencies. In addition, it is only too easy for you to sink just a little further into idleness, so that your fitness level drops even further. Fortunately, you can easily get above this base line if you are aware of it. Improvements can be made if you are willing to constantly look out for small ways in which you can take just a little more exercise than is strictly necessary.

As in all important matters, this is essentially a question of having the right mental approach. You have to see the point and want to follow it through. Much has already been made of walking instead of driving and climbing stairs rather than using the lift, but there are more ways than just those in which you can, without engaging in formal exercises, push yourself further up the fitness graph.

Did you ever think of acquiring a large dog? Imposing a moral obligation on yourself, in this case to provide the dog with the exercise he so obviously needs and so enthusiastically enjoys, is a good way to boost flagging resolve in the early stages of your new life. Did you ever consider joining a golf club? You will astonish yourself at the distances you walk, especially as a beginner, almost without noticing it, so occupied will you be with the physical and psychological problems of hitting the ball hard enough in the right direction.

Do you ever think about your posture? How do you stand? How do you walk? Do you *look* healthy? If you have a tendency to stoop, resolve right now to correct it, whatever your age. Slumping while standing or sitting, is an idle yielding to gravity, a refusal to face a challenge and beat it. It takes muscular action to stand or sit upright, and the muscles you need are probably in pretty poor shape. Postural defects are among the commonest causes of backache and may even lead to a 'slipped disc'. You can cure this by strengthening the muscles around the spine, but it is a great deal easier to prevent it by using the same means.

Watch a small child in action. Note the tremendous energy turnover, the constant movement, the marvellously comprehensive muscle usage and the wonderful flexibility in every joint. It is a simple fact that this degree of efficiency and flexibility *can* be maintained throughout life. It seldom is, of course, for a variety of reasons which include loss of interest in the physical use of the body as we get older. Those who maintain such interest – lifelong practitioners of Yoga, for instance – often maintain the same childlike range of body usage.

Try to remember this and apply it in your daily life. Do not do things only when you have to. Stretch, bend, twist at every opportunity. If necessary, *make* opportunities, not only to burn off a few extra calories but also to keep the range of joint movement you had as a little child. Remember too, that there is a pretty close correlation between the state of the body and the state of the mind.

Features of a good exercise plan

You will find plenty of keep fit manuals in the bookshops with details of exercise programmes. The differences between these is less a matter of the content than of the extent to which they provide good motivation by proper background explanation, and the care with which the exercises are graded so as to ensure build up of capacity without risk of injury. That apart, exercise schemes should be as efficient as possible in ensuring you achieve the desired result in the minimum time and should deal with as wide a range of muscles as possible. Unbalanced development is perfectly possible and although it is unlikely to cause grave problems, it is far from desirable.

Advancing years bring limitation of joint movement, mainly because of a failure to put joints through the full range of their articulation. This leads to loss of elasticity or even contracture of joint capsules. The resulting stiffness sets up a vicious cycle. Violent attempts to increase the range of movement in a short time are really asking for trouble and can cause life-long pain. Any respectable exercise programme must address itself to the need to increase and maintain mobility and must necessarily involve plenty of bending and twisting. It must also do this in such a graded manner as to preclude injury of any sort. At the same time, undue complexity is counter-productive. You should be able to memorise the routines quickly and should not have to exercise with the book in one hand.

Surprisingly, one of the best exercise plans available goes back so far that it almost certainly antedates anything comparable in print. This is the scheme of exercising worked out by the Canadian Air Force authorities in the 1950s expressly to meet the needs of people like you. People short of time, leading a generally sedentary life, and not too keen on displaying their unfitness in public. The 5BX, 11 minute a day plan for men and the XBX, 12 minute a day plan for women, meet all the requirements abundantly well.

The plan is excellently graded and you need never have any concern about dangers. Not, that is, if you read and stick to the rules and conscientiously follow the rate of progress as prescribed.

This plan is deservedly popular. Having been used in the Royal Canadian Air Force from 1958, it was published by Penguin in 1964 and has since been reprinted well over twenty times. The plan will certainly suit you, whatever your standard, as it ingeniously caters for all fitness levels from the barely tottering to the champion athlete. The book called *Physical Fitness*, is designed for both men and women and includes a short but useful introduction to each.

10 Health Farms

As a hard-headed executive, you are unlikely to believe that a week or two at a health farm is going to change your life. But this is not to suggest that health farms can offer no benefit – far from it. The idea, in principle, is excellent. Those that are well run and organised along lines with a sound medical basis are likely, given your co operation, to do you a power of good.

Heavily stressed executives like you, and maybe your spouse too, may very badly need a break from the endless competitive challenge of work. No matter how engrossing your work may be from time to time it becomes imperative for you to let go. It is hardly necessary to mention that the wives of highly successful men with enormous demands on their time, have a hard time too.

No doubt you do, from time to time, recognise the need for a period of change. So what do you do? Do you go to some tropical spot where you lie all day on a beach soaking in skin-destroying ultra-violet light? Lounge all evening in a bar or restaurant, stoking up with fortified drinks to give you the appetite to overeat expensive, unhealthy food?

Certainly you need a change, relief from pressures, relief from controlled aggression. You need a little pampering, rest and exercise, to be politely but firmly taken in charge. Where better to find it than at a well run health farm. Somewhat expensive, maybe, but certainly better for you than a sustained orgy of self-indulgence on the Cote D'Azur.

The medical element

Health farm management are beginning to recognise the commercial advantages of real medical back up and there is a tendency to delete 'farm' and substitute 'clinic'. Happily, you will not usually find a clinical atmosphere. Luxury is the order of the day and the medical ambience is deliberately low key. Clinical facilities are sometimes surprisingly extensive, but are kept in the background. These places are usually set in beautiful surroundings, with delightful views of lush countryside, and this kind of peaceful ambience is most beneficial.

Obviously, the emphasis varies from place to place and you must decide what it is you want. Do not expect any particular or immediate health advantage in a stay of a week or two. What you *can* get is a good health assessment programme, carried out without hurry and, being part of the rest cure, without your thinking that time is being wasted.

For example, Champney's have a fitness assessment routine using a bicycle ergometer test with heart monitoring which includes checks of blood pressure, respiratory capacity, height, weight, and an estimation of your body fat percentage. They also have a Well Woman programme with health discussions, cervical smear test and routine breast examination for cancer. There, you can also have a more complete medical check including full medical examination, X-rays, laboratory blood tests, etc. An excellent idea!

On the therapeutic side, some establishments have a major line in physiotherapy, with the accent on impressive machinery delivering a variety of forms of radiation, such as ultra violet, infra red or laser light, shortwave diathermy, ultrasound, faradic (pulsed) or galvanic (DC) electricity and so on. Unless you have an actual orthopaedic problem, you would be well advised to avoid such treatments. Even if you do need such treatment, a health farm is not really the place to have it.

Alternative therapy

You will no doubt already have a clear idea of what the medical establishment thinks of 'alternative medicine'. However, it would be unbalanced and unfair to the practitioners of the many forms of 'therapy' to suggest that these methods are wholly without therapeutic value. Alternative medicine flourishes for the cogent reason that, very often, it works. And it works for much the same reasons that orthodox medicine used to work in the days before we had antibiotics, beta blockers and steroids.

It was the very absence of effective therapeutic techniques that in the past made doctors so concerned with their patients and so apt to have a good 'bedside manner'. Knowing there was little they could do to modify the course of an illness, they were apt to modify their behaviour. Perhaps some would transmit confidence to their patient. More probably, they would feel genuine concern and express it by sitting down with the patient, holding their hand and wrestling with the crisis. All this created a good effect and often worked.

Therefore, do not be too dismissive of health farms which offer various forms of massage and other procedures involving physical touch. After months of repressed aggression and mental isolation in your work, you may find it therapeutic to be the recipient of a little well-meaning human contact. Massage is one of the oldest palliative treatments known to man and is undeniably soothing and relaxing. Claims that it increases the circulation in muscles and improves tone are doubtful, but its psychological value is undeniable.

Some establishments offer osteopathic manipulation to resore full and painless movement to joints and some osteopathic practitioners are very skilful in isolating and correcting minor joint problems. Manipulation is, however, sometimes dangerous and it is important to ensure that a proper diagnosis is made before treatment is given. Cases have occurred in which urgent medical treatment for a major

disorder has been dangerously delayed because the osteo-
path was not familiar with the condition and its signs.

Saunas, Turkish baths, steam cabinets, seaweed baths,
herbal baths, and so on are readily available and are all very
pleasant and enjoyable. However, you can safely ignore
claims that these experiences rid you of unspecified 'toxins',
'poisons', 'waste matter' or other unpleasant but wholly
imaginary substances. Wax baths are impressive and popular. To be painted from head to foot with melted wax, which
is allowed to harden, and then to be wrapped in silver foil,
plastic sheets and blankets and exposed for twenty minutes
to infra red light must surely have some kind of therapeutic
effect on the body.

You may, if you are so disposed, indulge in reflexology,
aromatherapy, vacusage, hydrotherapy, homeopathy or any
one of a host of other fringe activities. Do so, by all means,
but do not expect them to change your life.

Diets

In general, health farms can be relied upon to get the diet
right by offering a wide range of cereals, vegetables and fruit;
a moderate amount of boiled fish, poultry, cheese, yoghurt,
legumes and nuts; and hardly any fatty meat, butter, sugar or
oil. Some make much of the importance of medical examination before dieting, and purport to provide medical prescription of individual diets. Such offers need to be viewed objectively, since many health farm visitors could probably
endure a week of complete starvation with very little harm
and the suggestion that individual 'patients' require individually determined diets is questionable. Watch out for
diets that claim miracles of slimming. They are unlikely to do
you any harm in a period of one or two weeks, but equally
they are not going to do you any good. Even if you do lose
weight, you cannot keep them up and you will soon revert to
your old habits.

As explained in Chapter 8, the only object of diet amendment is to establish new and smaller eating habits. However

well chosen the diets at health farms may be, you are unlikely to achieve this desirable end in a week or two. But you can make a start under ideal conditions. If you can only keep it up afterwards, much will have been achieved and your money will have been well spent.

Exercise and sport

Although you are unlikely to be dragooned into bestirring yourself, you may well find that subtle pressures are put on you to participate in regular exercise sessions and to make use of the sporting facilities available. This emphasis on physical activity is excellent and, once again, there is the possibility that you may initiate new lifestyle habits.

Organised exercise sessions, if you can be persuaded to take part, may give you the motivation you need to try a little harder. There are sure to be people in worse shape than you. Do beware of the risks of sudden violent overactivity for joints have probably stiffened and ligaments lost their elasticity. Go gently at first and work up very gradually; heed the advice in Chapter 9.

Perhaps more attractive is the possibility of renewing acquaintance with sports you may not have engaged in for years. In the race for business or executive success you may have forgotten the pleasures and satisfactions of tennis, golf, squash, swimming, even walking. Now that you know how important it is to maintain your fitness, you may find the opportunity offered irresistible. Many health farms provide professional coaching in sports like tennis, swimming and archery and, of course, every golf course has its professional.

Beauty treatment

The most important aid to beauty is cleanliness and the achievement of a high standard of health. Many health farms also feature special beauty programmes with a wide range of treatments for body and face. These include solarium tanning (do not forget that the browner you are now, the older and more wrinkled you will look later on in life), depilatory waxing, skin packs and other facials of all kind, hair-dos, make up classes, and so on.

If you are a female executive, a quest for beauty in the context of health and fitness, may be the very thing you need as a relaxation after months of hard work. Executive wives, too, will need little persuasion to share the benefits of a health farm with their husbands, if these facilities are on the menu.

Prices

These vary considerably and when you consult the brochures, remember that VAT is to be added and that many invisible 'extras' are likely to swell the reckoning. Champney's, who prefer to be known as the International College of Health and Beauty, are at the top end of the scale with fees varying from £420 to £735 per week. At the other end the charges at the Tyringham Clinic, in Newport Pagnell, start at £116 per week. A Champney's Medi-check will cost you £160.

Typical charges for sports coaching, such as tennis, swimming and archery, are £10 to £15 an hour. Beauty treatments may come a little more expensive – waxing, £32 for both legs; solarium, £18; aromatic spa bath, £31; cathodermie bust treatment, £18, or £80 for five sessions; vacusage skin suction, £10. The choice is yours!

11 Psychosocial health

The promotion of health is not an end in itself, any more than your determination to achieve success as an executive is an end in itself. What you are really concerned about is personal happiness and that has been the main theme of this book. Health care matters to you primarily not because you fear pain or death, but because you know how poor health can interfere with your chances of happiness by curtailing the ability to live life to the full.

One of the central factors in personal happiness is the state of your psychological health and the way it affects your relationships with others. Any book of this kind would be incomplete without a consideration of the nature of psychosocial health and some prompting of your ideas on how to achieve it. Among other things, you must consider how you relate to other people and whether your performance promotes stable and mutually satisfying relationships.

Psychological health consists in the proper functioning of the thoughts, the emotions and the will. There is no clear borderline between the normal and the abnormal in any of these three divisions. It is all a matter of degree. All of us have, from time to time, been seriously mistaken in our thinking, but we do not believe that everyone is against us. You may often be a bit low in your spirits, but you do not plunge into suicidal depression. You may occasionally lack energy and drive, but are unlikely ever to reach the stage of mute, stuporouse idleness and withdrawal exhibited by the catatonic schizophrenic.

In your normal day to day life, at home and in the office, you may occasionally react with anxiety or pessimism, blaming others for the cause of your upset. You may experience real or imagined fears, especially in relation to your seniors, and may be tempted into petty criticism. Occasionally you may feel unjustifiably depressed, perhaps about your true abilities, and may resort to censorious comments about others.

These responses, even if infrequent, are damaging to your relationships with others, sometimes seriously damaging. Your personality determines to a large extent how far you tend to respond in these ways and it is very difficult for you to modify what seem natural responses. However, if you wish to be spared unhappiness, you must look very carefully at the way you relate to other people. It is the various aspects of such relationships that this chapter deals with.

As in the case of physical health, we start with widely varying degrees of handicap. Some of us are born with a hereditary disadvantage or have suffered early, damaging environmental influences. It may be that the effect of these can never wholly be overcome, and these influences can be entirely outside our control. Others can be blamed for your present difficulties and short-comings and you may consider 'throwing in the towel'. On the other hand, you can take the positive approach and resolve to make the best of the material you have to work with. In spite of the pervasive effect of these early influences, you can do much to improve the state of your psychosocial health. Equally, as in the physical context, much of the psychological ill-health you suffer is self-inflicted.

Psychological normality

As already mentioned, abnormality is easier to define than normality, but a look at the ideal case can be helpful. The notion of mature psychological normality is a very useful one. It involves most of the components of mental and social health and also points to the direction in which you should be striving. The ideal general characteristics possessed by the mature, psychologically healthy personality are:

(1) a capacity for, and constant engagement in, clear thinking,
(2) a controlled, but deep, emotional life,
(3) an effective determination to act,
(4) self-sufficiency in all ordinary matters, and the ability to manage affairs effectively,
(5) reliability and trustworthiness,
(6) a determination always to meet obligations in full.

Such people avoid getting into debt. They have a social conscience and are willing to play a part in ventures requiring co-operative activity. In their work they make a contribution to society and are not concerned solely with their own advantage. Work is important to them and they take much satisfaction in it. They have a reasonably accurate perception of themselves and will neither over-estimate nor under-estimate their own abilities. They accept the world as it is and try to make the best of it. Their personalities contain no grave self-contradictions. They are achievers. Their tendency is to look outward rather than inward, they show a proper concern for others and are able to relate easily to them. They are respected and liked by all to whom they relate.

Such paragons are, of course, rare but most of these qualities may, with effort, be cultivated and there is no reason why you should not strive after this kind of maturity. Do you think the effort worth the trouble? Read the above passage again, this time pondering on whether the possession of these characteristics would be likely to promote your happiness. If you agree that they would, consider how far you fall short of the ideal, and read on.

Censoriousness and self-preoccupation

A common indicator of psychosocial disorder is the habit of adverse criticism and fault finding. The springs of this trend are obvious enough. Each censorious comment contains the implicit statement, 'Of course, I am not like that!' and this brings the appropriate gratification. Business relationships are seldom intimate enough for censoriousness to do more than dent the *amour propre*, but the habit is deeply damaging to closer personal relationships. It has been the cause of an immense amount of disruption of friendship and marriage. Blaming others is undoubtedly comforting, but it is a comfort which may cost us dear and should be carefully avoided.

When the occasion for criticism is obvious, silence can earn respect, especially from the discriminating. Criticism of an absent third person is also an unendearing trait, for it invites the hearer to participate. Breaking the habit of gratuitous censoriousness is, for a number of reasons, a major step in the avoidance of unhappiness.

Adverse criticism, however, is sometimes justified. You, the executive, will occasionally, as a matter of disciplinary duty, need to apply verbal sanctions and even the behaviour of those close to us may have to be criticised. Always try to see things from the other person's point of view before commenting and, when appropriate, be careful to recognise the similarity of your own faults. Criticism, when applied, must always be relevant, accurate and specific. Too often, our response to the behaviour of others is merely one of general condemnation, which only has the effect of provoking aggression.

Honesty about feelings

Be as honest as you can with yourself and with others, especially in any close relationship. This is not always easy. Love and affection can vary with the changing circumstances of a relationship and open discussion is necessary. Honesty and the expression of affection can turn dislike into love. Be careful never to feign affection. Some people do so simply out of kindness of heart and a disinclination to hurt feelings. Some find it impossible to reject the advances of others, and allow

themselves to be drawn into a false position almost by iner-
tia.

Good relationships are amongst the greatest sources of
happiness and should be cherished as precious. They are,
almost by definition, based on honesty. So, if you want to
maintain them, be honest with the people you love.

Comparison with others

Man, especially executive man, is a hierarchical animal who
is deeply sensitive to his place on 'the ladder'. He sometimes
forgets that there are hundreds of different ladders and his
place is different on each. There are hierarchies of social position, physical strength, intelligence, knowledge, formal
qualification, wealth – the list is endless. Each of us sits
somewhere different on each of these individual ladders of
merit. The point is, of course, that wherever you may be
positioned on a hierarchy, there will always be those who sit
both higher and lower than yourself. Also, however high
you think you sit on one particular ladder, there will be
plenty of other ladders on which your position is lower.

To compare yourself with others, for the purpose of self-
approval, is delusory and pointless. It is not being suggested
that you should not strive to better yourself, but that you
should at all times have a realistic and suitably humble
attitude to your achievements. Comparison should be with
your own previous efforts, achievements or effectiveness,
rather than with the successes or failures of others.

Liking people

This can sometimes be difficult, and increased knowledge of
our fellow men does nothing to improve matters. The mistake is to assume that there are absolutes of character and
behaviour. This sort of naivety of opinion has been responsible for much social damage and unhappiness. People regularly have an effect on others which is simply a reflection of
the attitudes of the person making the judgement, usually on

the basis of inadequate information. It is not unusual to find that someone we dislike on first acquaintance, turns out in the end to be an admirable person. The change is not in that person's character but in their response to us. In the crowded and competitive world of business we are apt to look on others as rivals or threats, and this will inevitably condition our attitude to them and their response to us.

So, if you can somehow discover the good in people and express it, you will often find that they turn out to be much more congenial than you originally suspected.

Neurosis and hypochondria

A great deal of what is called 'neurotic' illness is really just imaginary. Much of it is consciously calculated to manipulate others and achieve some advantage. You must, however, recognise that many people who behave in this way have been unfortunate in their upbringing and have had more than their fair share of difficulty in coming to terms with the problems of life and human relationships. Some may be in need of reassurance and may crave affection, but be incapable of expressing the need except in the ineffective manner they have chosen. Some are profoundly afraid but unable to face their fears directly, or to recognise or analyse the causes of them.

It is questionable whether most 'hypochondriacs' are to be wholly acquitted of responsibility for their own unhappy state. Most people with this disorder have become more interested in themselves and their problems, than in the outside world. This is often harmful to the happiness of others who have to relate to them and are forced to come to terms with their unremitting self-absorption. The emotional needs of those who live with them are often neglected.

Anything which turns the attention of such people outward will be helpful, but an attempt should be made to understand the significance of the complaints which are of such interest. This is especially true of persistent physical complaints which have defied medical investigation. Here, an attempt should always be made to discover their origins. Did a parent or close relative die of cancer? Is there a concealed symptom which is causing secret worry? Remember that 'neurotic' people are not immune to organic disease. Many a doctor has been shocked to find a physical cause for a symptom he has been dismissing as 'neurotic' for months.

Mild hypochondriasis is one thing. Real neurotic illness is quite another. It would be naive to suppose that severe neurosis can be cured by even the most sympathetic and supportive help. Usually there is a fundamental defect of personality, arising during childhood, when the sufferer failed to develop the normal degree of fortitude and resistance to the vicissitudes of life. So severely neurotic people require a great deal of support and protection. They demand quite exceptional patience and understanding from those who have to live with them.

Attitude to work

It is not at all fanciful to suggest that our bodies and minds were designed for work. Work is, after all, simply the repetitive use of our faculties, whether physical or mental. These faculties arose, in the course of evolution, in response to an external need for their use. So work of whatever kind, should be regarded as an opportunity to use your mind or body for those things designed to maintain them in good working order.

It is because of this that work, appropriate to your ability, properly performed, invariably brings satisfaction. But the words 'properly performed' must be emphasised. Whether work is simple or complicated, it can be done well or it can be done badly. Skimped, hurried and careless work, got through as quickly as possible, brings no satisfaction, leads to loss of self-respect and incurs blame.

The enjoyment of leisure

The person who takes pride in the quality of his work, often adopts the same attitude to leisure activities. The well-motivated person will work as hard at leisure activities as at the daily job. Unfortunately, the common pattern is often one of poorly performed daily work followed by entirely passive 'leisure'. Purveyed entertainment of an entirely passive and non-participatory kind is a poor substitute for the lively and refreshing leisure use of the mind or the body. Even reading is preferable to passive TV watching and is more satisfying in the end, for at least active participation is involved.

Some little time must, of course, be spent in wholly passive relaxation. However, the natural counterpoise to hard work should not be to spend long evenings lying in a cosy armchair watching TV with a drink to hand. The counterpoise should be an engrossing leisure time activity affording refreshment and contrast and providing, if possible, as real a challenge as the main employment. Your day should be so filled that you look forward to sleep with pleasure. The refreshing, deep sleep of the justifiably tired, in which the mind and the body are restored.

So here are the seven basic rules for mental health:

(1) Look outwards rather than inwards.

(2) Avoid censoriousness.

(3) Avoid hasty judgements of people.

(4) Be honest with yourself.

(5) Do not compare yourself with others.

(6) Enjoy your work.

(7) Make the most of your leisure.

In the end the choice is yours. Hopefully, this book will have started you thinking along new lines to a fitter, healthier more fulfilling life, both professional and personal.

Glossary

ADRENALS Endocrine glands situated on top of the kidneys. They secrete various hormones, especially adrenaline and cortisol, which are required in time of stress but which may also have dangerous effects.

ALLERGY A reaction of the immune system to the presence of a substance to which it has been sensitised. Shows itself by skin rashes, tissue swelling, asthma, etc.

AMINO ACID One of the main constituents of protein. Two or more amino acids link to form polypeptides and these join to form proteins. Certain amino acids are essential for health.

ANATOMY The structure of the body. The study of the structure.

ANGINA PECTORIS A severe, disabling condition caused by inadequate blood supply to the heart. Exertion causes chest pain which may radiate down the left arm, through to the back or up into the neck. Angina results from atherosclerosis of the coronary arteries.

ARTERY A blood vessel carrying blood under pressure from the heart to the tissues. Healthy arteries are elastic and with smooth linings.

ATHEROSCLEROSIS A disease of the lining of arteries which may lead to thrombosis and blockage. Much of this book is concerned with the avoidance of atherosclerosis, which is the commonest cause of death in the Western world.

AVERSION THERAPY A form of treatment for alcoholism in which drinking is deliberately associated with unpleasant experiences.

AIDS Acquired immune deficiency syndrome. A virus disease with a very high mortality in which the normal immunity to infection and certain forms of cancer is lost as a result of the damage caused to 'T' lymphocytes by the HIV (human immunodeficiency virus).

BILE A fluid formed in the liver, stored in the gall bladder, and passed down the bile duct to the intestine where it acts to emulsify fat taken in the diet, so that it can be absorbed.

BILIRUBIN Formed in the liver from haemoglobin. A constituent of bile. Its retention in the body, in liver disease, causes jaundice.

BLACK STOOLS If bleeding occurs high in the intestine (as in stomach or duodenal ulcer) the blood is altered and appears jet black when seen in the stools. An important sign which should never be ignored.

BRONCHOSPASM Narrowing of the bronchial tubes in asthma or bronchitis.

CALORIE The heat required to raise one Kilogram of water by one degree centigrade. One Calorie is equal to about four Joules.

CARBOHYDRATE The main constituent of most diets. Bread, potatoes, sugars and rice are mainly carbohydrate. Glucose, the principle fuel of the body, to which carbohydrates are broken down, is a monosaccharide. Starch, and other complex carbohydrates, are polysaccharides (polymer chains of simple sugars).

CARBON DIOXIDE The waste gas given up by the tissues and breathed out in the lungs.

CARBON MONOXIDE A very poisonous gas found in cigarette smoke and car exhausts. Forms carboxyhaemoglobin in the red cells and reduces the ability of the blood to carry oxygen.

CARCINOMA A cancer of surface cells. The commonest class of cancers. Cigarette smoking causes carcinoma of the lining of a bronchus in the lung. This is called bronchial carcinoma.

CARDIAC ARREST Cessation of the normal heartbeat.

CEREBELLUM The smaller, lower and subsidiary part of the brain, concerned with control of balance and movement.

CEREBRAL THROMBOSIS One of the causes of 'stroke'. The blockage of a small artery in the brain. Always serious because important body functions, such as movement, speech, understanding, sensation, etc. may be affected.

CEREBRUM The main part of the brain.

CHOLESTEROL A fatty steroid, essential to health, but dangerous in excess. One of the elements laid down in the lining of arteries to form the atheromatous plaque of atherosclerosis.

CHRONIC Lasting for a long time. From the Greek 'chronos' which means 'time', as in 'synchronous' or 'chronometer'.

CHRONIC BRONCHITIS Persistent cough with production

of sputum. Commonly caused by smoking. May lead to the more serious condition of chronic obstructive airway disease.

CIRRHOSIS OF THE LIVER A serious disease in which a network of scar tissue forms throughout the organ, replacing normal liver cells and interfering with its function.

COMPUTERISED TOMOGRAPHY CAT scan, or CT scan. A valuable and improved form of X-ray investigation in which the data from a large number of separate, narrow-beam exposures are reassembled by computer to form a detailed image.

CONGENER The ingredients in alcoholic drinks which confer the identity. Congeners contribute to the hangover, making brandy and port more 'heady' than gin or vodka.

CORONARY ARTERIES The first tributaries of the main artery of the body, the aorta, just as it emerges from the heart. The coronary vessels form a 'corona' or 'crown' for the heart, branching and supplying the heart muscle with the substantial blood supply which it needs to continue beating.

CORONARY THROMBOSIS An obstruction to the flow of blood in a coronary artery or one of its branches. This is almost always the result of atherosclerosis. The part of the heart muscle supplied by the blocked artery dies and the seriousness is determined by the size of the branch concerned.

CORTISOL The natural steroid hormone produced by the adrenals. The drug 'Cortisone' is identical, but has now been superceded by a range of more powerful cortico-steroids.

DELIRIUM TREMENS A severe mental upset caused by withdrawal of alcohol in a chronic alcoholic. Features vivid, terrifying hallucinations and delusions.

ENZYMES Protein substances which accelerate biochemical reactions. Many different enzymes operate throughout the body. Essential to life. Enzymes like 'pepsin' and 'trypsin' act on food in the bowel to break it down to absorbable compounds.

ETHANOL Ethyl alcohol. The essential ingredient of all alcoholic drinks.

GLUCOSE The essential fuel of the body. All carbohydrate eaten is converted to glucose.

HAEMOGLOBIN The substance in the red blood cells which links to, and transports, oxygen.

HORMONE A chemical messenger released into the blood and causing an important effect elsewhere in the body. Putuitary hormones control the other hormone-secreting (endocrine) glands.

HYPERTENSION High blood pressure.

HYPOCHONDRIASIS The unreasonable and unsubstantiated conviction that one is suffering from an illness.

INSULIN The hormone of the pancreas which controls blood glucose levels. Its absence or deficiency causes diabetes.

JAUNDICE Staining of the skin with bilirubin when the latter cannot pass through the liver into the bile. A grave sign in cirrhosis of the liver.

KAPOSI'S SARCOMA A cancer which was rare before AIDS victims began to show the condition.

LIFE-LONG OBESITY An abnormal increase in the number

of body fat cells, occurring in childhood as a result of over-eating, and persisting throughout life.

LOCOMOTION The function of movement from place to place, effected by the muscles, operating on the bony skeleton.

MENINGIOMA A benign tumour of the brain linings.

MUSCLE Contractile tissue which brings about movement of the skeleton and some of the soft tissues.

OLFACTORY Relating to smelling.

OVARY The source of the ovum and of the hormones controlling the menstrual cycle. Usually one ovum released per month.

OXIDATION The process of combining with oxygen and releasing chemical energy.

OXYGEN The most vital of all bodily requirements. Stoppage of the supply for more than a few minutes is fatal.

PANCREAS The source of important digestive enzymes and also of the hormone, insulin.

PEPSIN The main digestive enzyme of the stomach, breaking down protein.

PERISTALSIS The process whereby food is passed along the inside of the bowel. Smooth circularly-placed muscle fibres contract behind the bolus of food and relax in front of it. This goes on continuously, right along the length of the bowel.

PHYSIOLOGY The study of the functioning of the body.

PROSTATE GLAND A gland surrounding the urethra, just

below the bladder, which secretes part of the seminal fluid. Enlargement with age is common and this may lead to obstruction to the outflow of urine.

PROTEIN One of the main building substances of the body and an important constituent of the diet. Muscles are made mainly of protein.

ROUGHAGE Unabsorbable material in the diet, usually cellulose. Helpful in avoiding constipation.

SARCOMA A malignant tumour of tissues other than surfaces.

SMOKING The principle avoidable hazard to health. Responsible for millions of deaths each year. Smoking has been clearly implicated in cancer of the lung, mouth, tongue, stomach and bladder, as well as in heart disease and high blood pressure.

STRESS The body's response to the awareness of a need for a greater than usual effort. Can become a source of illness.

STROKE Cerebral thrombosis or haemorrhage.

THROMBOSIS The clotting of blood in an artery or vein and its consequent blockage.

URETERS The tubes which carry urine from the kidneys down into the urinary bladder.

URETHRA The tube from the bladder to the outside for the passage of urine. In the male, it also carries seminal fluid.

UTERINE TUBES Sometimes called 'fallopian tubes'. They carry the ovum from the ovaries to the uterus. Fertilisation, by spermatozoa, usually occurs in the uterine tube.

UTERUS The womb. There, the fertilised ovum embeds itself, forms the placenta, and grows into a foetus.

VAS DEFERENS The tube carrying the spermatozoa from each testicle to the seminal vesicle on its own side. A permanent form of contraception (vasectomy) involves cutting or tying these tubes.

VEIN A low-pressure vessel carrying deoxygenated blood back to the heart from the tissues.

VITAMINS Essential substances which must be provided in the diet if health is to be maintained. Very small quantities are required and excess provides no advantage.

Useful Addresses

Alcoholics Anonymous
11 Redcliffe Gardens
London SW10
Tel: 01-352 9779

ASH (Action for Smoking & Health)
5/11 Mortimer Street
London W1
Tel: 01-637 9843

British Cardiac Society
2 Beaumont Street
London W1
Tel: 01-486 6430

British Diabetic Association
10 Queen Anne Street
London W1
Tel: 01-323 1531

British Heart Foundation
102 Gloucester Place
London W1
Tel: 01-935 0185

British Lung Foundation
12a Onslow Gardens
London SW7
Tel: 01-581 0226

British Medical Association
Tavistock Square
London WC1
Tel: 01-387 4499

British Rheumatism & Arthritis Association
6 Grosvenor Crescent
London SW1
Tel: 01-235 0902

BUPA
300 Grays Inn Road
London WC1X
Tel: 01-278 4651

City Health Care
4-7 Chiswell Street
London EC1Y 4TH
Tel: 01-638 4988

Health Education Council
78 New Oxford Street
London WC1A 1AM
Tel: 01-631 0930

Occupational Health Management Ltd
324a King Street
Hammersmith
London W6 0RF
Tel: 01-741 5022

Private Patient Plan
Tavistock House South
Tavistock Square
London WC1H 9JE
Tel: 01-388 2468

Royal College of Physicians
6 St Andrew's Place
London NW1
Tel: 01-487 3414

Royal College of Surgeons
35 Lincoln's Inn Fields
London WC2A
Tel: 01-405 3474

The Sports Council
16 Upper Woburn Place
WC1H 0QP
Tel: 01-388 1277

The Chest, Heart & Stroke Association
Tavistock House North
Tavistock Square
London WC1H 9JE
Tel: 01-387 3012

Weight Watchers (UK) Ltd
11 Fairacres
Dedworth Road
Windsor
Berks
Tel: Crawley 35571
01-508 9148

Western Provident Association Ltd
Culver House
Culver Street
Bristol BS1 5JE
Tel: 0272 273241

155

Index